W9-CCY-374

THE PALEO
VEGETARIAN
DIET

THE PALEO
VEGETARIAN
A Guide for Weight Loss
and Healthy Living
DIET

Dena Harris

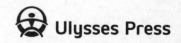 Ulysses Press

Text copyright © 2015 Dena Harris. Concept and design copyright
© 2015 Ulysses Press and its licensors. All rights reserved. Any
unauthorized duplication in whole or in part or dissemination of this
edition by any means (including but not limited to photocopying,
electronic devices, digital versions, and the Internet) will be prosecuted
to the fullest extent of the law.

Published in the US by:
Ulysses Press
P.O. Box 3440
Berkeley, CA 94703
www.ulyssespress.com

ISBN13: 978-1-61243-443-8
Library of Congress Control Number: 2014952013

Printed in Canada by Marquis Book Printing

10 9 8 7 6 5 4 3 2 1

Acquisitions editor: Katherine Furman
Managing editor: Claire Chun
Project editor: Alice Riegert
Editor: Lauren Harrison
Proofreader: Renee Rutledge
Layout: Lindsay Tamura
Index: Sayre Van Young
Cover design: what!design @ whatweb.com
Cover artwork: front © stockcreations/shutterstock.com;
    back © Pichest/shutterstock.com

Distributed by Publishers Group West

NOTE TO READERS: This book has been written and published strictly
for informational and educational purposes only. It is not intended to
serve as medical advice or to be any form of medical treatment. You
should always consult with your physician before altering or changing
any aspect of your medical treatment. Do not stop or change any
prescription medications without the guidance and advice of your
physician. Any use of the information in this book is made on the
reader's good judgment and is the reader's sole responsibility. This book
is not intended to diagnose or treat any medical condition and is not a
substitute for a physician.

For anyone who has struggled with food. I hope this book makes it an ally versus an enemy.

Contents

A Note from the Author

I had been a vegetarian for 20 years when I decided to give Paleo Vegetarianism a go. No beans. No soy. No dairy. No rice. No quinoa. No alcohol (um, yeah…we'll talk). No grains of any kind. And, obviously, no meat. Friends thought I was crazy. And for a while, I agreed. I mean, just what was a MorningStar breakfast patties addict like me supposed to *eat*?

My decision to try a Paleo Vegetarian diet came when I met a number of health-obsessed people eating Paleo and experiencing phenomenal results. Like the type A skeptic I am, I started researching Paleo and Primal diets and was intrigued by what I found. I started a website about my Paleo Vegetarian journey and was amazed at the response. It turned out that I wasn't alone. Tons of vegetarians, it seems, are interested in the benefits of a Paleo diet.

The biggest obstacle—obviously—is that consuming meat is at the heart of any Paleo diet. So what are a bunch of plant eaters supposed to do?

Answer: Go Paleo—only without the meat.

It wasn't easy. That means no beans, soy, rice, dairy, alcohol, or added sugars? That pretty much wiped out every recipe I'd ever made as a vegetarian.

But eating Paleo Vegetarian *can* be done. This book is a tool to get you started. Pay attention to what you eat and how you feel, and you'll quickly learn what parts of the diet do and don't work for you. Once you learn the basics, you can make adjustments. Maybe you're okay with the occasional inclusion of rice or beans. Maybe you find a bowl of morning oatmeal before a hard workout does you no harm. This will thrill some of you and make others cringe, but there are no hard-and-fast rules that apply 100 percent of the time—in life and especially in a diet. Instead, what's here is a foundation upon which you can build.

It's taken almost 30 years of dieting—and being heavier than I should be for most of that time—for me to get to a point where I feel like food is my friend and not an enemy to be combated, outmaneuvered, and outwitted at every turn. Making the switch to include Paleo eating in my life has been a big part of this mental switch. I hope what's outlined in these pages will do the same for you.

Some thank-yous are in order. If it takes a village to raise a child, it takes an army of understanding friends and family to see a writer through the draft of a book. To say I ran around frazzled would be a kind understatement. So a huge and heartfelt thank-you to all friends, family, and coworkers who were patient with me, calmed me, believed in me, and reminded me to feed my cat when I grew distracted.

In good health and good spirit,

—Dena

Part I

What Is Paleo Vegetarianism?

Chapter 1

Paleo Vegetarian Health Benefits for Weight Loss and for Life

Paleo Vegetarian? Uh…isn't that an oxymoron? Kind of like "decaf coffee"? Aside from the fact that it doesn't exactly roll off the tongue to anyone with even a little bit of knowledge about the Paleo diet and vegetarianism, the pairing makes no sense. *Sooo… You're a vegetarian who follows a primarily meat-eating diet? Uh-huh. That doesn't seem like it would be a problem. At all.*

Fair enough. But the fact that it's a marriage of opposites doesn't negate the fact that multitudes of hardcore, in-it-for-life vegetarians are interested in exploring the possibility of adapting their diet to the Paleo lifestyle. Some, like me, came to the idea through the CrossFit phenomenon that has swept across our nation. Reading and witnessing how many of these super-strong, super-lean athletes were transforming their bodies through Paleo made a number of us do a double take and say, "Hey—I want that for me!" Others are hearing and reading more about the damage grains are doing to our bodies and wondering if there might be something to the notion of grain-free living. Still others are stymied by weight loss and baffled as to the cause behind their weight gain or inability to shed pounds.

Why Adopt a Paleo Vegetarian Lifestyle?

First of all, let's agree to call it "PV" for short. For vegetarians reading this book (and I assume most of you reading this book *are* already vegetarians, otherwise you'd be looking at a traditional Paleo diet), the "V" part of the equation is likely something with which you've already come to grips. Whether for moral, ethical, environmental, or a combination of reasons, you're clear on why you choose to eschew meat. This leaves the second part of the equation to be answered: Why are you interested in adhering to a Paleo diet?

Before jumping into Paleo, let's pause to examine the word "diet." It's a term fraught with emotion. For many of us, it conjures up memories of grapefruit and fiber, "replacement meal" shakes, and countless hours spent tracking and recording every morsel of food that went into our mouths. (Ask any woman over 30 the caloric value of anything from a frozen fruit smoothie to cream cheese brownies and she'll be able to spit out the answer before you can say, "Weigh in.")

Yet for all the fad diets, all the Weight Watchers and Jenny Craigs and days spent eating fat-free treats and low-sodium rice cakes, we're still not where we want to be. We yo-yo up and down on the scale. We surround ourselves with guilt around food. We give up on our goals, thinking they're unrealistic, too hard, or too far out of reach.

And maybe they are. Other than teenagers in love, there is no one as self-delusional on the planet as a would-be dieter. We know—

know—that once we lose the weight our love life will improve, we'll get a better job, redecorate the house, become a more patient parent and altruistic spouse, volunteer to help the homeless on weekends, write the novel that's been percolating inside our brain for the last ten years, and transform into the 5'10" natural blonde we were born to be. (Never mind that we're a 5'4" shaggy brunette and medical science has yet to document the spontaneous growth of six inches of toned legginess to any physique, no matter how many desserts you say "no" to.) Dieters, God love them, are probably the most optimistic people on the planet.

However, optimism and reality don't always occupy the same space. For that reason, I would encourage anyone starting this or any eating plan to understand what exactly it is they're after *before* they sauté the first vegetable.

Why is this important? I had an obese friend declare to me, one day out of the blue, "I'm eating nothing but small salads and working out twice a day until I lose 80 pounds!" And you could tell from her enthusiasm that in the moment she said it (sitting on her couch as we watched TV), she meant it.

As you would expect, her commitment to perfect health lasted less than 48 hours. There was a crisis at work that required long hours and, just like that, "Nothing will stop me!" was shelved for "I'll try again later when I'm not so busy."

Sound familiar? My friend's goal was optimistic, but not realistic. I'm an exercise enthusiast known around my office as the "Food Nazi" for my adherence to healthy eating, and even I wouldn't have lasted three days on my friend's plan. You have to take into account life and balance.

Runners spend a lot of time talking about fast-twitch and slow-twitch fibers. These are the muscle fibers that give a sprinter short, explosive bursts of power (fast-twitch) or marathoners and century cyclists the endurance to carry on aerobically for long periods of time (slow-twitch).

All of us are born with a pretty even mix of fast- and slow-twitch fibers, but most people find they're better at one type of activity than another (i.e., sprinting as opposed to running half-marathons). This is largely due to genetics. While muscle fibers can be trained (within reason) to convert, say, a fast-twitch sprinter into a long-distance runner, we each have a natural propensity toward excelling at one type of activity over another.

I bring this up to make the point that as much as we may want to make losing weight and gaining health a fast-twitch push, we'd do better to realize that dieting is about activating our slow-twitch mental muscles. We need to take a deep breath, focus, and settle in for the long haul.

Adding in Paleo: Ask Yourself What You're Hoping to Achieve

Setting a goal is not the main thing. It is deciding how you will go about achieving it and staying with that plan.

—*Tom Landry, National Football League coach*

Declaring, "I want to lose 20 pounds," is not the same as having a realistic plan you can follow to lose the weight. Saying, "I want to be toned in every inch of my body" with no working knowledge of weightlifting is not going to create lean muscle, no matter how much you may wish it so.

So the question before you is, where do you want to be? By following a Paleo Vegetarian diet, what is it you're hoping to achieve?

Yeah, okay, I hear you all screaming, "We want to be thin!" Thank you, *Cosmo*, for making every woman over a size four feel unworthy as a human being. I get it. Few people pick up a book with the word "diet" in the title solely to explore better health. And there are certainly weight-loss opportunities to be found within these pages. So if you're here solely for the weight loss, that's okay. As Socrates said, "Know thyself." But I hope as you work through this book that you'll embrace other reasons, such as the ones listed below, for eating Paleo Vegetarian.

- Sustained weight loss

- Eating whole, natural foods

- More energy and stamina

- Better sleep

- Reduced bloating

- Mental clarity and improved mood

- Increased fitness levels

- Fat burning versus sugar burning

- Reduced allergies

- Lowered risk for diabetes, heart disease, and cancer

- Feeling confident and in control of your diet, yourself, and your life

Eating Paleo Vegetarian offers the opportunities for all these things. I'm reminded of one of my favorite Facebook posts that circulates from time to time. It shows a "skinny-fat" woman (thin appearance but no muscle tone) and the caption reads, "This woman weighs 130 pounds." Next to her is a picture of a smoking hot, completely ripped woman, the kind whose body most of us dream of having. The caption here reads, "This woman weighs 145 pounds." Then underneath both pictures it asks, "Who would you rather look like?"

The point is that when most people say they want to lose *weight*, what they really mean is they want to lose *fat*. Many, many people transform their bodies on a Paleo or Paleo Vegetarian diet without huge weight-loss numbers. There's a big difference between a healthy and lean 150-pound frame and a bloated and saggy 150-pound frame. Same number, different body. Frankly, my advice is to throw away your scale. Now. Seriously, toss it. I haven't owned a scale for over ten years. "But wait," you say. "Without a scale, how will I know if the diet is working?"

You'll know. Measure inches or how you look and feel in your clothes. Or start counting the "You look great! What's your secret?" comments you'll soon be receiving.

Scale, schmale, people. It's just a number. Don't let it dominate your life.

Getting Real: Your Reasons for Eating Paleo Vegetarian

I promise—this isn't one of those touchy-feely books that asks you to write down the emotion you experience every time you eat a grape. Other than a fun quiz in a bit—in which you can choose to participate or not—this is the only writing-required portion of the book, so please play along.

In the spaces that follow, write down three reasons for wanting to try the Paleo Vegetarian diet. Be as specific (and realistic) as possible, but do not list a specific weight-loss goal. Instead, strive for statements such as "I will feel comfortable in my clothes and confident in my appearance." Limit your range to one to three goals so you don't overwhelm yourself. Remember, as you achieve goals, you can always go back and add new ones.

1. _____

2. _____

3. _____

How will you know when you have achieved these goals? You might say, "I'll know I've achieved the goal of being confident in my appearance when I can: wear a sleeveless T-shirt/wear my shirt tucked in/tighten my belt buckle a notch/accept a compliment because I think someone means it and they're not saying it just to be nice."

1. _____

2. _____

3. _____

What is your timeline for achieving these goals? Remember— slow-twitch!

I will reach goal number 1 by _____.

I will reach goal number 2 by _____.

I will reach goal number 3 by _____.

What are some unrealistic expectations of which you may need to rid yourself? Example: "I'm going to lose 20 pounds and completely transform my body in one month."[1]

1. _____

---

1   Not to burst your bubble, but no, you're not. Here's a good test: If upon hearing your goals friends either laugh *or* give you a pitying look and place a hand on your shoulder and say, "Of course you will!" you may not have set a realistic goal.

2. _____

3. _____

Whom can you count on to support you in your pursuit of adhering to a PV diet? This is important. You want to surround yourself as much as possible with people who truly believe in you, who understand that this is a lifestyle choice and not a "fad diet," and who won't engage in subtle sabotage, i.e., "Can't you cheat on your diet just this one time?" These people are hard to find, so think carefully. Then make an extra effort to engage these people in your life over the next several months. List names below.

1. _____

2. _____

3. _____

4. _____

5. _____

Oooh...you did so well! You answered all the questions! Ha. Kidding. I know you just read through everything and made a halfhearted promise to come back later and fill them in. Cheating already, huh? I'm on to you. Consider this the first test of your commitment to the PV diet. Put the book down, go find a pencil or pen, come back, and answer the questions above. You can do it—I believe in you!

Heads Up: It's Easier to Be Vegetarian Than It Is to Be Paleo

I used to laugh a silent laugh when meat eaters (did anyone else refer to them as "muggles" during the Harry Potter frenzy?) or pure Paleoists would look at me and say, "I don't know how you can be a vegetarian. I think it would be so hard not to eat meat."

The truth is—and most of you know this—being vegetarian in today's world isn't all that hard. Here's why.

REASON #1: MORNINGSTAR, BOCA BURGERS, AND AMY'S KITCHEN

In 1988 I was living with my parents outside Dayton, Ohio, preparing to enter college. On more or less a whim, I decided to go vegetarian for 30 days. I never once missed meat, and while I never intended to stay vegetarian, the thought of eating meat after the 30 days were up was enough to turn my stomach. My 20-plus-year voyage into vegetarianism had begun.

I'm not sure about other parts of the world, but at least in rural Ohio in the late '80s, not eating meat was not looked upon favorably. Raised eyebrows, pursed lips, etc. There was also the question of *what* to eat. My meatloaf-loving Midwestern parents had no idea what to serve me other than pasta with plain marinara sauce. As a college student, beer[2] and pizza were my go-tos. After college I moved to a small (pop. 3,500) town in North Carolina where I was suspected of being an atheist, hippie, and potential communist, all because I didn't eat meat. The manager of our local grocery store literally thought I was making up a vegetable when I asked if his store could please carry edamame. As for prepared vegetarian meals, the freezer case held nary a soy burger in sight.

Change came eventually and life grew easier, for me and numerous other vegetarians. Being able to pop a "burger" in the microwave or make a quick sandwich from soy deli meats and soy cheese

---

2   Don't judge me. This was before Google so there was no way to know most beer was nonvegetarian.

was a delicious luxury. And it led to the second reason being a vegetarian today isn't all that hard.

REASON #2: PEOPLE ARE MORE ACCEPTING

With everyone from movie stars to your local librarian shunning meat, being a vegetarian is no longer seen as operating outside the social norm. Even die-hard meat eaters are forgoing meat with at least two to three of their meals each week. I have to think not being made to feel "weird" or like an outcast has opened up the door to many more people exploring the options of a vegetarian lifestyle.

REASON #3: A LINE IN THE SAND

For many—but not all—vegetarians, there is simply a moral line most won't cross. Again, from the first moment I declared myself vegetarian, I was never tempted to eat meat. It was simply something I wouldn't do. I never had to exert willpower to remain faithful to a vegetarian diet—especially once I educated myself about the treatment and processing of animals for the majority of meat consumed in this country. Now, eating a *healthy* vegetarian diet is something entirely different, and that did take some time and getting used to. But not eating meat? No-brainer.[3]

I haven't had the same experience with eating Paleo. I still struggle on occasion with the decision not to eat grains, soy, rice, and dairy. Maybe it's because I don't picture sad cow eyes when the urge to eat a bowl of cereal hits. It also strikes me as unfair that wanting to chow down on some Moroccan couscous—something I used to tell myself was healthy—is now off-limits.

---

3   This is not true of everyone. I have numerous committed vegetarian friends who admit they still find it hard to live without bacon, and who look longingly at a steak while eating their braised tofu salad.

The bottom line is that while the muggles of the world wonder at the willpower required not to eat meat, most vegetarians would agree that when you have your reasons firmly in place for why you're choosing not to eat meat, fish, and/or dairy, it's easier to stay the course. It doesn't mean the desire to eat meat may not still be there for some, but it's easier to stay behind that hard line you've drawn in the sand and not stray.

Choosing to Eat Paleo

So let's translate that mindset to the Paleo Vegetarian diet. What can we do—what can *you* do—to draw that mental line in the sand that says, "I choose to eat this way because I want to. Not because I have to, not because I'm forcing myself to, not because I think this is the only avenue left for me to lose weight and I'm desperate, but because this is the choice that makes sense for me, my life, my values, and how I choose to live and exist on this planet."

Eating PV will be easier and become a lifestyle if you are clear upfront about why you're making these choices. There's nothing wrong with admitting you're eating PV as a trial, or simply as a short-term measure to lose weight. If anything, telling yourself the truth will make it easier for the duration you decide to stay in. Personally, I know I'm more likely to stay committed to something—anything—if I know I'm only in it for a limited duration.

"Hold the squat for 30 more seconds. You can do anything for 30 seconds!" says my trainer at the gym. It's the same thing with starting a new diet regime. Set your time frame and commit to it. Decide to eat PV for one day. You can do anything for one day. Then go for one week. You can tough anything out for one week. If that works for you, try two weeks. Then a month, and so on.

Where I don't want you to falter is by declaring, "Starting tomorrow, I shall eat Paleo Vegetarian from now until the end of time!" and then instantly regret the decision as soon as you crave ice cream. Although it may not always come across, I am a believer in balance. And if you tell me I can never, ever eat pizza, ice cream, or a slice of my Aunt Jo's hot-from-the-oven apple turnovers sprinkled in powdered sugar ever again…? Well, game over people.[4]

I'm guessing it's the same for you. You may try to eat PV for a day or two, but the eternal enormity of what you've undertaken will get to you sooner rather than later, and you will fail the diet and the diet will fail you. I'd prefer that *not* happen. So what's the solution? Keep reading.

Why Can't I Just Stay Vegetarian and Lose Weight?

I like a world of absolutes. Eat this, not that! Do this exercise and watch that muscle develop! Up is up and down is down!

Unfortunately, there are few absolutes in life and the "good/bad" argument for almost any way of eating can be made. The fact is, most diets out there will get you weight loss—IF you're able to follow them. That "if" is the downfall of many of us. We're a nation that enthusiastically embraced the liquid diet once we saw Oprah lose the weight. But none of us—including Oprah—could stick with it. I personally haven't tried a lot of the rogue diets, but I've read that even eating a diet of nothing but, say, cereal or an all-fruit diet will shed the pounds. Once again, this probably works only if you're able to stick to the diet's limitations, with what I would

---

4   Can you eat all these things and still stay lean and healthy? Yes, with caveats. We'll cover that in Chapter 8: Cheat Days and the 80/20 Principle.

imagine is a drastically reduced calorie count. You'll lose weight on an 800-calorie-a-day diet of candy, but who can live like that?

Still, most people appear to be of the persuasion that eating a vegetarian diet is a good way to lose weight. I suspect that's because most people assume vegetarians are super healthy, but, as we've discussed, that's not always the case.

Once I started paying attention to people who did eat a seemingly *very* healthy vegetarian diet—low fat, whole grains, lots of fruit—I noticed something. These weren't the super-slim people of the world. In fact, most of them had girth, especially in the belly area. And what I saw happen body-wise to the children of a close friend truly made me start questioning the value of a vegetarian diet based on grains.

My former yoga instructor is a lifelong vegetarian, one of those granola people who converted when she was ten. She and her husband—a meat eater—have three kids, three years apart in age. Everyone was impressed by the diet regime of these kids. Voluntarily, they refused soda when it was offered to them. They snacked on cauliflower and fresh cherry tomatoes. They requested tofu for dinner. They loved couscous and bulgur and sprouted-grain bread. They were the models of healthy eating.

And yet.

I moved away from the town where my instructor taught but reconnected with her several years later via Facebook. At this point, her kids were probably 13, 10, and 7 in age. And when I saw pictures of the kids, my jaw dropped. All three of them were huge.

This is not due to apathy. These kids are involved in football and dance and soccer and all sorts of sports. The family is active and goes hiking and camping on weekends. I can't imagine anything happened where my friend suddenly broke down and started feeding her kids fried food. And indeed, her Facebook page is filled with links to the vegetarian (all heavily grain-based) meals she's preparing each week.

My takeaway is that grains are bloating the hell out of these kids.

I've watched other friends go through a similar experience. Several of my running friends attempted a vegetarian diet only to abandon it less than a year later because, even with all the running, they kept gaining weight. These are disciplined people running 50 miles a week—and they kept going up on the scale once they became vegetarians and replaced meat with grains.

Obviously this is a highly biased and unscientific sample, but my belief is that grains, soy, and dairy—but especially grains—are toxic to our bodies when ingested in large amounts. And most every vegetarian I know bases his or her meals on grains. I do think that the 80/20 principle, making sure we're only ingesting a bit of the bad with a steady diet of the good, is the most effective way to feel healthy, look good, and lose weight. Using this rule as a guideline (see Chapter 8), most any food can have a place in our lives.

Chapter 2

How PV Do You Want to Be?

At one point in my life, for eight months, I went vegan. Even before that though, when I was a vegetarian who eschewed all meats and seafood but still indulged in honey, eggs, and cheese, I was pretty intolerant of vegetarians who weren't as devoted as me. Call it snobbery or elitism, but I refused to recognize that cutting red meat out of a diet but still eating chicken, turkey, and fish counted as being a vegetarian. Or, my favorite, a coworker who told anyone who would listen how much better she felt since she had switched to a vegetarian diet, but who could be counted on to order a hamburger every time we went out to lunch. (When I finally asked her about it, she explained to me that she was a vegetarian except for the times she ate meat. Swear to God.)

Even as I was looking down my nose at others, I recognized the hypocrisy of my actions. I personally came to vegetarianism in stages. For the first five years, the only foods I gave up were red meat and pork. Then—against the pleas and wishes of my then husband—I ditched chicken and turkey. After eight years of that, I gave up fish, sometimes wavering on whether or not shellfish counted.[5] I finally abandoned all fish and, for a brief time, made the jump to vegan.

Vegan was hard for me. I simply didn't have the moral boundaries with eggs and honey as I had with thighs and wings. Chickens were going to lay eggs and bees were going to make honey whether I partook of them or not. I did stand behind the moral argument that the *manner* in which most consumer eggs and honey are collected from animals are, in a word, appalling. But when our neighbors up the street offered us fresh eggs from their chickens, Trudy and Lunch,[6] and I could pick up honey at our local farmer's market from a man who, stating it mildly, LOVED his bees, I found my interest in being vegan waning.

These days, I'm much more of the mindset that everyone is doing the best they can. It's none of my business if someone is religious about sticking to their no-meat pledge or if they use it as a fluctuating guideline. Just as it's no one's concern if I still enjoy the occasional wheat- and sugar-laden bagel as a treat. (And for the record, oh yeah, I do.) My life, my rules.

Of course, reasonable people will disagree. I'm all in favor of educating people on the atrocious conditions animals in this country endure, but my hard-earned experience over the years is that in-your-face preaching and condemning does little to change people's actions. What *does* get people's attention is looking healthy, having energy, and enjoying an active life. Combine

---

5   I pretty much decided it counted unless someone set a big ol' platter of lobster or crab legs with a side of hot butter in front of me. Then it didn't count. Hmm. Maybe I have more in common with my old coworker than I realize...

6   Trudy and Lunch were much-loved pets and pampered, to boot, with a chicken crib that would not have been out of place on *Lifestyles of the Rich and Famous*. They also loved to be held and petted. Nothing cracked me up more than seeing my neighbor go into his yard and call out, "Here Lunch, here Lunch!" and watch this affectionate chicken come running.

that with being willing to engage in reasonable, nonaccusatory conversations about diet choices and the reasons you chose to eat the way you do, and you have the makings of the type of conversations that can change minds and change lives.[7]

With that being said, just as there are different types of vegetarians, so too are there different levels or types of Paleo eaters. Where do you fall on the ladder? To help you decide, let's do a quick, cursory overview of the variations found in both camps. We'll start hardcore and work our way back to the more flexible options.

Different Types of Vegetarians

VEGAN: The bane of chefs everywhere, vegans are nonetheless the badasses of the vegetarian world. Aside from no meat, fish, or fowl, most (but not all) vegans also forgo the use of animal products such as leather or silk.[8]

LACTO VEGETARIAN: No meat, fish, fowl, or eggs, but cheese and dairy are acceptable.

OVO VEGETARIAN: I could never be an ovo vegetarian just because I think of the word "ovulation" every time I see the term and erupt in a disheartening array of elementary-school giggles. Ovo (hee-hee-hee) vegetarians are the ying to the lacto yang. They

---

7   As an aside, I'll share that the more I try to withhold information, the more people want to know. When asked why I didn't eat meat, I'd answer, "Oh, you don't want to hear me get on my bandwagon about that," and people who were standing with arms crossed would drop them and say, "No, I really would like to know." Or I'd say, "I won't go into details because it's pretty bad, but once I found out what laying chickens in this country go through, I just couldn't buy regular eggs," and they'd say, "Really? Like what?" Let the education begin.

8   So maybe I was never a real vegan. We owned leather couches and at the time I was vegan I recall I had a *smokin'* hot pair of leather high-heeled boots.

do not eat meat, fish, fowl, or dairy. They do, however, consume eggs.

LACTO-OVO VEGETARIAN: This is what most people mean when they say they're a vegetarian. No meat, fish, or fowl, but dairy, eggs, and cheese are okay.

PESCATARIAN: Considered by some to be "pseudo" or "semi" vegetarians, pescatarians do not eat red or white meat or fowl but live to dine out at Red Lobster. Kidding. But this group is okay with eating fish and shellfish.

POLLOTARIAN: Again considered by some to be "semi" vegetarians (but not us, because we're not here to judge people, right?) the pollotarian does not eat red meat, fish, or seafood. Instead, they consume only poultry and fowl.

There are, of course, people who don't fit easily into any group. For example, there was a brief time period when I didn't eat red or white meat or fish or cheese, but I did eat shellfish and eggs. Or there are people who for the most part stick with a plant-based diet but occasionally see nothing wrong with eating a hamburger if they're craving one. Some people refer to these mixed plant-based diets as "flexitarian," some don't consider them vegetarians, and some people who follow these mixed-vegetarian diets consider themselves full-fledged vegetarians.

As long as you have your own reasons straight in your head for choosing whichever path you're on, it really shouldn't matter if you fit directly into a single group or not.

Different Types of Paleoists

You may be surprised (or not) to learn there's a similar scale for people who practice a Paleo diet. The classifications aren't as defined or accepted as the vegetarian ones, but the trend is moving in that direction. For the purposes of this book, I've commissioned my own classification system.

HARDCORE: The vegans of the Paleo world, these are the people that follow a Paleo diet to the letter, including giving up all alcohol. All meat is grass-fed. All seafood is wild-caught. They buy their food in-season and do their best to live as our ancestors did on a true Paleo "caveman" diet. Would they go so far as to club their own meat and bring it back to their man cave (if that were an option)? Quite possibly, maybe.

PRIMAL: Mark's Daily Apple (www.marksdailyapple.com) is the bible of the Primal world and well worth reading even for those following a PV versus a traditional Primal diet. (The level of medical physiology on the site behind how what we eat affects our bodies is as well researched and impressive as I've found anywhere.) Primal differs from Paleo in that it allows for limited dairy, including small amounts of goat cheeses and full-fat products such as butter and heavy cream (good news for coffee drinkers!). Limited alcohol with a preference for red wine is also tolerated and even encouraged. Primal is also more relaxed about eating saturated fats from things like coconut oil and eggs. The biggest difference is that the Paleo diet is almost 100 percent about diet while Primal followers consider the guidelines they follow more of a comprehensive plan for living that includes getting enough sleep, small movements throughout the day, stress management, etc.

MODIFIED PALEO: Some people modify a Paleo diet to reach certain goals. For example, people looking to get lean will often rule out Paleo-approved starches such as sweet potatoes or squash due to the higher carbohydrate count of these foods. Some Paleoists avoid fruits for the same reason: high sugar count that works against weight loss. Some eat a hardcore Paleo diet but make an exception for wine or beer.

THE "MORE OR LESS" PALEOIST: This group eats a primarily Paleo or primal diet but leaves the door open for hedging. Some people follow an "80/20" principle (which we'll discuss in Chapter 8) where they eat Paleo or Primal 80 percent of the time but don't lose sleep if they eat a piece of Mom's apple pie or pancakes every now and again.

As you can see, just as there is no "right" or "wrong" way to be vegetarian, there is no "right" or "wrong" way to be Paleo. The hardcore Paleoists will, of course, argue that point, but I'm going to go back to the "my life, my rules" options. A diet won't work for you unless it *works* for you. If you demand sheer perfection of yourself but find you're slipping off the diet every day by 3 p.m. because it's just too hard, then that's not the right diet for you.

What Kind of Paleo Vegetarian Do You Want to Be?

So now we get to it. What kind of Paleo Vegetarian diet will you follow? The answer is probably already predetermined by where you are now with your level of vegetarianism, but it's worth taking a moment to consider your answer for this reason: You're going to be cutting out a lot of your regular protein sources on a PV diet. Successfully sustaining a PV lifestyle will be immensely easier if you eat eggs and fish or seafood of some kind. That being said, I don't want or expect anyone to give up on firmly held principles. If you're a lacto vegetarian, then chances are you'll be a Paleo-lacto vegetarian or a Primal-lacto-ovo vegetarian. That's a little cumbersome, however, so for the intents and purposes of this book, we'll stick with the PV title for everyone.

WHY MEAT-EATING PALEO
PEOPLE AREN'T THE ENEMY

I almost titled this sidebar, "Can't we all just get along?"

For the life of me, I can't understand why Paleo folks and vegetarians position themselves at opposite ends of the spectrum. I mean, okay, I *get* it, as meat is a big deal to both groups, for opposing reasons. But it turns out that we really aren't that far apart. We might not be ready for the group hug, but we're getting there…

Ask people what sort of person they think of when they hear the word "vegetarian," and most likely what will come is the image of…the hippie. Granola-loving, bell-bottomed, long-haired, peace sign–waving, carrying-spiders-out-of-the-house-instead-of-smooshing-them-with-their-shoe-like-normal-people hippies.

Would you say that's an accurate description of you and your vegetarian friends? I know for a fact that the "live and let live" vegetarian stereotype doesn't apply to me. I have a deal with all spiders, crickets, cockroaches, and ants: If I'm in their territory, out in nature, they have free rein to live long and prosper. The minute they cross the threshold of my condo, game on. I will squish a spider with the best of them. It's called survival of the fittest and I won't apologize. (I also wouldn't be able to sleep if I knew I let a big hairy spider scurry away in my bathroom when it was in my power to stop him.) Does this make me a lesser person? Maybe. But it also means I've never conformed to the "hippie" version of a vegetarian so many uninformed people carry.

By the same token, Paleoists do not fit the stereotype of chest-thumping, meat-worshipping carnivores. When I started investigating Paleo, I was *amazed* by how much Paleoists and vegetarians have in common. That's right, I said it.

The truth is, most true Paleoists, while obviously not eschewing meat, care a great deal about how the animals their meat comes from are treated and raised. They are as appalled by McDonald's burgers and Oscar Mayer deli slices (full of nitrates and preservatives) as any card-wielding vegetarian. Many of them refuse to eat any meat that doesn't come from grass-fed, humanely raised animals. Yes, there's still a seemingly irreconcilable difference between the two factions, but as a whole, I've found the Paleo world to be filled with people who express sincere concern and dismay for the current treatment of animals for commercial-meat purposes, and who refuse to participate in the buying chain.

Bean-Eating PV?

While I leave it up to you to choose the level of vegetarianism you'll engage in, I strongly suggest you abandon the hardcore Paleo plan, specifically for the reason that allowing some properly prepared beans into your diet will help form a non-animal protein base. Beans can go a long way in helping you find a quick and simple way to ingest some protein. It's not textbook, but you know what? Neither is not eating meat on a Paleo diet, and we're already breaking that rule so why not push the envelope? Besides, I'm willing to bet money the Paleo police don't show up at your door.

To wrap up, you'll notice in the recipe section that there are options for various levels of PV. Some of the recipes call for eggs or include fish or dairy, and several include beans. There are also recipes that are more stringently in line with a full Paleo Vegetarian hard-line diet. Modify as necessary to meet your PV needs. Remember, the reason you picked up this book is most likely because you want to lose weight in a healthy way, and there is nothing healthy about a lack of protein in a diet.

Chapter 3

A Primer on Why No Grains, Why No Beans (and Answers to Your Most Pressing Questions on Other PV Foods)

These days it seems as if everyone is jumping on the gluten-free train. Walk down any grocery aisle in America and you won't get more than two feet before your eyes are bombarded with an excess of gluten-free packaging. Everything from frozen waffles to protein bars dangle before us the glittering allure of a gluten-free world.

Gluten-free is not grain-free, however. To illustrate the point, remember in the '90s when America was in the grips of a fat-free frenzy, stuffing SnackWell cookies down our throats at an unprecedented rate? The overindulgence (ten cookies in a sitting instead of two) actually prompted something called "The SnackWell Effect," which is a term for how people go overboard when they think they're being given a free pass. We thought not having fat in our food was the answer, yet that was the decade when the American waistline seriously swelled up.

These days, we find ourselves in a similar situation with gluten. People read "gluten-free" and think they're home free. It's the SnackWell Effect all over again. Just because a food is labeled "gluten-free" doesn't make it nutritious. More importantly, it also doesn't automatically make that food Paleo-approved.

So what is Paleo and what are the guidelines? Below is a quick overview of the theories behind the most questioned "no grains/ no beans" rules of Paleo, as well as rationale and guidelines on other foods often questioned on the Paleo diet. This is not a comprehensive list or scientific study. It's a general overview to get you started. As you enter the world of Paleo, I recommend a deeper dive into the science behind why certain foods are encouraged and others banned. Understanding how food works in our bodies is especially helpful for some of the Paleo gray areas such as white rice, potatoes, and green beans. When you understand and pay attention to how your body reacts to these foods, you have the information necessary to decide whether or not to make them a part of your diet.

If you take away nothing else from this book, take this: In order to more easily lose weight—without feeling hungry— you want to become a fat-burning machine.

What's Wrong with Grains?

Let's start with the big one, the concept that makes would-be Paleoists cringe: no grains. Cereals, whole-grain toast and bagels, steel-cut oats, quinoa (quinoa!), and all our other favorites are suddenly forbidden. But why?

Grains contain gluten, which is a sticky, water-soluble protein found in cereal grains such as wheat, barley, and rye. But wait—gluten is a protein. Protein is good, right? So what's the problem?

The problem is that gluten is an inflammatory protein. It causes irritation to the gut lining and can lead to the not-so-pleasant sounding "leaky gut syndrome." In addition, grains such as wheat, barley, and rye contain antinutrients that prevent your body from absorbing the healthy nutrients you're feeding it.

In the Paleo world, you'll frequently hear grains referred to as "toxic." This is usually a reference to the phytic acid (aka phytate) also found in grains. Phytic acid is one of the antinutrients that prevent the proper digestion of food. Diets high in phytic acid, such as your typical American diet with its emphasis on whole-grain foods, cause mineral deficiencies by blocking the absorption of calcium, iron, copper, zinc, and magnesium.

Toxicity aside, when it comes to weight loss, grains are a serious inhibitor given their high carbohydrate content. When carbohydrates enter the body, they are broken down into glucose or sugar in the blood, creating a giant leap in insulin production. This insulin leap not only leads to "crash and burns" (think of the 2 p.m. slump you have at your desk after a big lunch), but your body will store any excess glucose as fat.

If you take away nothing else from this book, take this. In order to more easily lose weight—without feeling hungry—you want to become a fat-burning machine. *Fat burning.* Most everyone walking around eating the typical "healthy" American diet—even the skinny people—are sugar-burning machines. Burning fat instead of sugar holds numerous advantages, including:

- Sustained energy throughout the day
- Lack of carb/sugar cravings

- The ability to exercise longer and harder
- No need to "carbo-load" before a workout
- The ability to miss meals without getting cranky, hungry, or crashing

How do you burn fat instead of sugar? You reduce the amount of sugar you put into your body. As sugar and carbs typically go hand in hand, reducing the intake of one typically leads to reducing the intake of the other.

Here's the deal. The body can only store so much glucose, so it's not a dependable energy source. Also, when glucose is gone, that's when you find yourself ravenous. This creates a vicious cycle. Your body sends out cravings for carbs. You eat more carbs than you can store. The extra glucose created from the carbs is stored as fat. When you do exercise, the first thing burned is the small amount of stored glucose. This starts the cycle of hunger and carb cravings all over again.

When you're a fat-burning machine, your body holds onto its small store of glucose for as long as possible, burning through fat *first* and only getting to stored glucose if it's really needed, such as at the end of a high-intensity sprint workout. With your body looking to fat (instead of sugar) for energy, you'll miss out on those insistent hunger pains, making weight loss easier.

How do you know if you're burning fat rather than sugar? Your hunger levels are the easiest measurement. People who are fat burners can easily go for hours without feeling hungry. Missed meals are no big deal. Sugar burners, when they miss a meal, will feel the very real pangs of hunger—those stabs in the stomach that let you know it's time to eat, NOW. Fat burners may think food sounds good, but if they miss a meal those hunger pangs don't occur.

Another way to measure fat-versus-sugar burning is through your workouts. One of the biggest myths out there is that we need to eat a good meal or snack before we exercise. The truth is, most people aren't doing anywhere near the level of exercise they'd need to have their glycogen stores replenished by the copious amounts of carbs they're eating. If you can get up in the morning and work out on an empty stomach, or do a hard workout without carbo-loading or in a fasted state, congrats. You, my friend, are a fat-burning machine.

If you're not there yet, don't worry. The good news is you can train your body to become a fat-burning machine, and the Paleo Vegetarian diet does just that.

PSEUDOGRAINS

Vegetarians have a closer relationship to pseudograins than most people, so we often have a harder time giving these up. Amaranth, buckwheat, couscous, and quinoa are staples in our kitchens. And let's not forget other grains like spelt, triticale, Kamut, farro, and oats. And yes, even though these were pushed on us as being "power foods," they are all banned from the Paleo diet.

How do pseudograins differ from regular grains? Pseudograins are the seeds of broadleaf plants. Regular grains, by comparison, are the seeds of grasses. While these pseudograins are gluten-free (wait—make that GLUTEN-FREE!), they bring their own problems to the table, including chemical compounds that cause similar digestive and inflammation issues as cereal grains.

In addition, some of these grains (spelt, triticale, Kamut, and farro) still contain gluten. Oats are theoretically gluten-free but are subject to cross-contamination with wheat gluten from processing facilities. Oats also contain similar amounts of phytic acid as found in wheat, which, as we just learned, is a no-no. Bottom line? No grains.

Why No Beans?

If the lack of grains in a Paleo diet elicits the most sobs from carb lovers, beans run a close second, especially among vegetarians who see beans as the Holy Grail of protein.

"Why no beans? Beans aren't junk food!" exclaimed an indignant vegetarian friend when I explained the basis of the PV diet to him. He looked at me as if I'd just insulted his mother.

You can understand his outrage. It's easy to look at pizza crust as the enemy, harder to reconcile "lentil soup" as something harmful.

Let's first go broader in our understanding of "beans" and use the term "legumes." In the broadest sense, a legume is a bean, pea, lentil, or peanut. (That peanut part will become important when we get to the other Holy Grail of a typical vegetarian diet—peanut butter.) Beans don't contain gluten, so we're safe there. They do, however, contain phytates, the same antinutrient found in grains that prevents the absorption of healthy nutrients.

Like grains and pseudograins, beans are inflammatory to our systems. The quickest way to observe this is the gassy effect beans have on people. I used to joke that after 20 years as a vegetarian, I had a stomach of steel. I could eat a bowl of beans, follow it up with some eggs and still not have to excuse myself from the room. However, after following a Paleo diet and now eating only the occasional legume, I can see (bloat) and feel (gassy) the effect they have on my body.

Like grains, beans are also high in carbohydrates, making it a challenge to lose weight when large quantities are consumed.

Many vegetarians who favor beans over bread are puzzled as to why the weight sticks around. It's not just beans themselves, but it's the quantity we eat. Nuts also contain phytic acid, but most people aren't subsisting on a meal of almonds, so the few carbs and phytates they get from a handful of almonds aren't overly impactful. It's not unusual, however, to have a cup or more of pinto beans as a side dish or black beans as the base for the new vegetarian burrito recipe you just found. Beans deliver a wallop of carbohydrates because we eat them in mass quantity.

There's evidence that soaking, sprouting, or fermenting beans helps reduce the amount of phytates they contain. If you're following a PV diet for health and not weight loss, you may want to experiment and see how your system handles the inclusion of beans in your diet. Although high in carbs, beans do provide an easy source of protein. Just take care to read up on the processes available to break down the phytates before you consume the beans.

Commonly Questioned Foods

There are a number of non-Paleo foods that leave people scratching their heads. Are they allowed or aren't they? If so, how much? And if they're not allowed, why the heck not? Below we address some of the most frequently asked questions about common foods.

NUTS

As just mentioned, nuts contain phytic acid, that pesky inhibitor of healthy nutrients. In fact, nuts typically contain more concentrated levels of phytic acid than either grains or legumes. Say whaaaat? So why are nuts allowed while beans aren't?

In a word, quantity. Nuts are meant to be snacks. Eating ten almonds or cashews a day is a lot different from tucking into a big bowl of black bean tortilla soup.

There are two things to understand about phytic acid. One is that although it's often demonized, humans can tolerate phytic acid in small amounts, e.g., in a small serving of nuts. The other point is that phytic acid has to come in contact with minerals and nutrients in order to prevent their absorption. So, if you're snacking on nuts, the best thing to do is to eat them separately from other foods. Have a handful of almonds or a couple of macadamia nuts as a midmorning snack, but don't eat them with your meals.

SEEDS

Like seeds? You're in luck. Although edible seeds such as chia, flax, hemp, sunflower, sesame, and pumpkin pose some potential digestive and dietary problems, like nuts, they're generally eaten in such small quantities that it's not a big deal. So while you don't want to make seeds a mainstay of your diet, you can kick back and enjoy some sunflower seeds sprinkled in your salad or pepitas in your next Mexican dish. *Olé!*

CORN

When I was strictly vegetarian, I used to keep a bag of frozen corn handy just so I could sprinkle kernels into recipes for flavor and health. At least, I thought I was being healthy. Corn has recently become the whipping boy of the health food movement, and with good reason. Corn may technically be a vegetable, and it is gluten-free, but it's been so genetically modified that there's just no nutritional value left in it. It's also high in starch and therefore not good for weight loss. For these and other reasons, it's also not Paleo. So when someone passes you the corn, just skip it.

GREEN BEANS

Green beans are a legume so they're forbidden, right? Wrong! Green beans (and snow peas) are an exception to the rule. While technically a legume, they're very low in phytic acid and lectins, making them an acceptable Paleo choice. Cooking them reduces their phytic acid levels even more. In the role of side dish, few people find they have digestive problems with green beans. If you're one of these people, avoid them. Otherwise, fresh green beans in-season are chock-full of vitamin C, folate and, magnesium, so enjoy.

PEANUT BUTTER

A decidedly non-PV friend and her three-year-old toddler popped by for a surprise visit. When her son asked for a snack, she was dismayed to learn I didn't keep Cheerios, Go-Gurt, string cheese, or Goldfish crackers in the house.

"I forget you're not a mom," she said, laughing. "Whatever. Just hand me your peanut butter."

"Umm…" I said.

My friend rolled her eyes and gave a deep sigh. "No peanut butter? Seriously?"

Yeah, seriously. No peanut butter. Peanuts are a legume and contain phytic acid, lectins, and something called aflatoxins, which sounds kind of cute (like the Aflac duck), but which are actually toxins produced by a mold that grows readily on peanuts and is found in most peanut butters as well. Store-brand peanut butters are also filled to the brim with sugars and salts. If choosy moms had a clue, they would *not* choose Jif, or any other commercial peanut butter on the market. You may as well be feeding yourself and your kids teaspoons of straight sugar with that stuff.

A better alternative is almond butter, preferably fresh-ground, to avoid the added sugars, salts, and oils found in commercial brands. However, I warn you, a little goes a long way. Personally, I can't keep almond butter in the house. It's like a crack addiction. I'd sell my mother's wedding band to score some and, when I get it, I can't stop at a single serving. Instead, I enter a nut butter frenzy where I spread it on bananas and celery and dark chocolate and brussels sprouts (don't judge me) and look up only to find the jar I just brought home empty before it ever hits my pantry. My only comfort is that I'm not alone. Overindulgence of nut butters is an issue for many people—and a big inhibitor to weight loss. In fact, every time I start to gain weight I look at my nut butter consumption and realize I'm overindulging. My solution is to treat almond butter the same way I treat dark chocolate. It's a treat to be enjoyed occasionally without guilt, but not something I should be nibbling on at every meal.

RICE

You know how you're never supposed to discuss religion or politics? I'm adding the category of "whether or not eating rice is allowed on a Paleo diet" to that list. Life would be simpler if everything was black and white, but that's rarely the case. There are some strong opinions out there on this issue, and there is no right or wrong, so it will be up to you to decide where you'd like to land.

Let's start with the hardcore perspective. No rice. Rice is white, rice has little to no nutritional value, and rice is high in carbohydrates. Rice equals bad. *Unless…*

An alternate camp categorizes white rice as a "safe starch." While not claiming rice is good for you (i.e., offers health benefits), the rationale is that white rice is basically a gluten-free, empty carbohydrate with no toxins attached to it.

Notice the emphasis on white rice. It comes as a surprise to many people that white rice has more going for it than does brown rice—the beloved carbohydrate of the celebrity and dieting world. In fact, brown rice, while containing more nutrients than white rice, also contains more problematic elements, including what should now be the all-too-familiar phytate protein inhibitor. (Wild rice contains antinutrients as well.) Brown rice can be made healthier, but it involves more prep work (soaking, etc.) than most people are willing to do.

Here's where I come down on the issue. If you're seeking to lose weight, avoid it. Otherwise, a little white rice here and there in your diet is still Paleo-safe. As a sushi-fanatic, there's no way I'm giving up rice 100 percent. And I don't have to, so long as I'm not eating it with the majority of my meals.

OH BOY, NO SOY!

I know. I *know*. No soy is a blow. Best to just embrace it. Say bye-bye to soy burgers, soy cheese, soy hot dogs, soy milk, soy crumbles, soy sausage, soy nuggets, soy buffalo wings, and soy protein powder—and the list goes on.

You're probably sick of hearing the phrase "phytic acid" at this point, but guess what? Soy is really, really, *really* high in phytates. As a Paleo Vegetarian, you're already going to be challenged to fit in all your vitamins and minerals, and anything that blocks the absorption of calcium, magnesium, zinc, and iron needs to be on the "uh-uh, no thanks" list.

The other issue with soy is that the majority of it is genetically modified. Paleo Vegetarianism is about eating whole foods—real foods. While we don't have to break the bank and eat organic everything (more on this later), we should be cognizant of foods that have been altered so much they barely resemble the food they were originally based on.

Another strike against soy: It lists among the highest pesticide contamination of any crop. Phytoestrogens are another black mark against soy. Phytoestrogens, aka soy isoflavones, have been shown in some studies to promote the growth of tumors. There is also a concern that soy can lower testosterone levels in men. How bad soy is for you and if some soy is better than others remains an ongoing debate. Again, if you have questions and concerns, I encourage you to do a deeper dive into the myriad of reasons soy is banned on the Paleo diet. Know, however, that to follow the PV diet outlined in this book, soy is excluded. The occasional handful of edamame (young soy beans still in the pods) won't kill you, but for the long haul, avoid all soy products.

OILS

I remember my collection of cooking oils from back in the day when I was a vegetarian. I had them all—canola oil, safflower oil, corn oil, sunflower oil, peanut oil, grapeseed oil. Every time I found a recipe that called for a new type of oil, I was delighted.

If your kitchen currently resembles what mine used to look like, you'll need to ditch the highly processed vegetable and seed oils in your cabinet. (I know, grapeseed oil isn't cheap. Throw it out anyway.) Make sure you toss *all* vegetable and corn oils, as well as soybean oil and seed oils. When I first went Paleo, I assumed seed oils were okay but have since learned they are exceptionally high in omega-6 fatty acids and best avoided, as alternative oils are available. In fact, there are an abundance of healthy oils that all fit the PV plan. The list of oils includes the Paleo go-to, olive oil, but also nut oils such as almond, walnut, macadamia, and sesame oils, as well as avocado oil, hazelnut oil, and butter or ghee.

You'll see in many recipes that coconut oil is the darling of the Paleo world. The reasons for this are many. Coconut oil is low in polyunsaturated fat and holds up well under high heat. (Roast some green beans drizzled in coconut oil—you'll thank me.) The health claims for coconut oil range anywhere from supporting the immune system to boosting metabolism (and promoting weight loss) to helping to reduce sugar cravings and improving the health of your scalp. Magic elixir? Maybe, maybe not. But it is healthy, and the smell and taste is pleasing to a majority of people. Coconut oil is now my go-to. I even spread it on my Paleo toast in place of butter and ghee.

ALCOHOL

For all the hardcore pure Paleoists I've come across—and having been a member of CrossFit, I've come across quite a few—I have rarely met one who held to the Paleo rule of no alcohol. (Before you get all smug, let me point out that I also have run across a number of hardcore vegetarians in my day who have been more than willing to turn the other cheek when it came to drinking their beer of choice that may or may not have been vegetarian-approved.)

Don't get me wrong—the Paleo teetotalers are out there. And they have my admiration. My unscientific opinion is that giving up alcohol is probably a good thing for our bodies—the poor food choices that come with imbibing is reason enough.[9] But as Prohibition proved, we like our drinks. And the good news is that you can eat PV and still enjoy a reasonable amount of adult beverages. Reasonable being a glass or two occasionally.

Robb Wolf, one of the gurus of the Paleo world, recommends what's known as the "NorCal Margarita." This is a drink popular

---

9   Or, wait—is that just me?

among Paleoists and something you may want to check out. Being Paleo Vegetarian throws a twist into presenting a definitive list of what alcohols are and aren't PV-friendly. For example, red wine is the go-to alcohol of choice for most Paleoists as it contains the fewest carbs and additives. But some wines contain gelatin or caseins, products some vegetarians prefer to avoid. Beer contains gluten and is, sadly, not Paleo-friendly and also generally not vegetarian-friendly, as animal products are sometimes used in the filtering process. When it comes to PV guidelines on alcohol, I recommend three principles:

1. Do your homework ahead of time. You know what you like to drink, so Google it and figure out if it meets PV guidelines. If it doesn't, decide whether you're okay with that.

2. Practice moderation.

3. For weight loss, avoid alcohol. It's empty calories, and again, it's amazing how often having even just one social beverage can lead to poor food choices.

Embracing the Paleo Vegetarian Lifestyle: The PV Quiz

Still with us? Impressive. So let's dig a little deeper. Take this quick quiz to determine why you want to live the Paleo Vegetarian lifestyle and where some of your strengths and challenges lie.

1. I've been a practicing vegetarian for:
   a. Less than 5 years.
   b. 5 to 10 years.
   c. Over 10 years.
   d. I'm still a vegetarian if I only eat meat sometimes, right?

2. I became interested in the Paleo diet through:
    a. The extensive reading I've done.
    b. Friends.
    c. CrossFit.
    d. This book is the first time I've heard of it.

3. The hardest thing for me about being a vegetarian is:
    a. Getting enough protein.
    b. Not being able to eat what my friends and family eat.
    c. Nothing—it's not that hard.
    d. All the damn cooking that's involved.

4. The best part for me about being vegetarian is:
    a. I feel like I'm staying true to my morals.
    b. Eating a lot of vegetables.
    c. I like being different from everyone else.
    d. I love feeling healthy.

5. I was able to transition to being a vegetarian:
    a. In stages.
    b. Slowly—I backslid a couple of times.
    c. Quickly, all in.
    d. I still struggle with remaining 100 percent committed.

6. I think sugar is:
    a. Delicious.
    b. Like most things, fine in moderation.
    c. Evil.
    d. Wait. Where are you going with this?

7. On average, each night I get:
    a. 7 to 8 hours of sleep.
    b. 4 to 6 hours of sleep.

c. Less than 4 hours of sleep.

d. Huh? What? Sorry, I was sleeping.

8. I'm willing to spend time each day cooking and preparing food.

    a. No, but instead I spend time once a week prepping food for the week.

    b. Yes, unless there's something really good on TV or I'm tired or it's a Tuesday and then no.

    c. Yes.

    d. No.

9. The opinions of family and friends about my diet and what I eat:

    a. Are important to me.

    b. Matter to me, but I don't believe them to be as educated as me about diet and health.

    c. Don't matter to me.

    d. I wish everyone would just mind their own business.

10. I am a stress eater.

    a. No.

    b. Yes.

    c. I would be if I allowed myself, but I have self-control.

    d. Why else do people eat?

11. I'm interested in changing my diet to Paleo Vegetarian:

    a. To lose weight.

    b. For my overall health.

    c. I love a challenge.

    d. A lot of my friends eat Paleo.

12. When it comes to willpower and diets I would say:
    a. My willpower comes and goes, depending on how my day is going.
    b. I try not to get too stressed or obsessed if I eat something not on my diet.
    c. I am a rock. Give me a plan and I'll follow it.
    d. I struggle with not eating the things I want.

13. I think most diets:
    a. Would work, if people would follow them.
    b. Are unnecessary. People should just learn to eat better.
    c. Offer a way to mix things up so people don't get bored.
    d. Are hard to follow because there's not enough food allowed.

14. The most important thing to me is:
    a. Finding an eating plan that works for me and that I can follow for life.
    b. Being healthy.
    c. Feeling like I have control over my diet and cravings.
    d. Being thin.

15. I want to add the Paleo aspect to my current diet because:
    a. I keep hearing about how great everyone feels on a Paleo diet and I want to try it.
    b. The reasons for not eating grains, beans, and dairy make sense to me.
    c. People say it can't be done.
    d. It's a quick fix to lose weight.

16. I plan on eating PV:
    a. Slowly at first, maybe building into it by excluding grains for a month, then pseudograins, then beans, etc.

b. As a test at first. I'll decide whether or not to continue after I see how I feel and what my results are.

c. As a challenge, just to see if I can do it.

d. For the rest of my life.

17. The hardest thing for me to give up on a Paleo Vegetarian diet will be:

    a. Pasta in all it's many, lovely, enticing forms.

    b. Bread for sure.

    c. My morning oatmeal.

    d. Everything. This is going to suck.

18. I have a history of starting and stopping diets.

    a. I don't diet so much as I modify my eating based on new information I learn.

    b. False.

    c. Most diets I've done have worked for me. I just get bored so I intentionally switch it up.

    d. True.

19. I believe the Paleo Vegetarian diet will work for me because:

    a. I understand the principles behind why certain foods are prohibited. It makes sense to me.

    b. I'm not sure it will.

    c. I'm willing to put in the work.

    d. I'm desperate.

20. I think the biggest mistake people make with their diet is:

    a. Not spending enough time researching to see if the diet makes sense.

    b. Expecting too much, too soon.

    c. Not having enough willpower to see it through.

    d. Cheating.

21. Most of the popular diets on the market:
    a. Have elements in them that make sense but don't work in my current vegetarian (or other) lifestyle.
    b. Are unrealistic.
    c. Would work if people would follow the plan.
    d. Are only there to sell books and make money.

22. I would describe my exercise routine as:
    a. Simple and consistent.
    b. Eclectic. I'm always mixing it up and trying new things.
    c. It's *on*, dawg. I bet I can do more push-ups than you.
    d. Yeah, about that. I'm planning on starting my exercise routine any day now…

23. If people mock or laugh at my way of eating, I will:
    a. Address their concerns but do my homework so I have answers to their questions.
    b. Roll my eyes and make a note to avoid talking about food and diet with them in the future.
    c. Ignore them and let them wallow in their Cheetos-eating misery.
    d. Challenge them to a cholesterol test.

24. Which of these diets have you tried? Select all that apply.
    - ❑ Weight Watchers
    - ❑ Jenny Craig
    - ❑ Richard Simmons (Hey now—showing our age!)
    - ❑ *The Biggest Loser* diet
    - ❑ Slow Carb
    - ❑ The Mayo Clinic Diet
    - ❑ South Beach
    - ❑ Atkins
    - ❑ Body for Life
    - ❑ Cabbage Soup Diet
    - ❑ Nutrisystem
    - ❑ Slim-Fast
    - ❑ Sonoma
    - ❑ Wheat Belly
    - ❑ The Zone
    - ❑ Dr. Oz

- ❏ Dr. Phil
- ❏ Dr. Andrew Weil
- ❏ Eat Right for Your Body Type
- ❏ Raw Food Diet
- ❏ Cookie Diet (Seriously, people?)
- ❏ Best Life Diet
- ❏ Kind Diet
- ❏ Other

How did you do? Count the number of "a," "b," "c," and "d" responses to see how well suited you are to enter the land of PV.

MOSTLY A's: THE PLANNER

You'll read the research and buy the book, but you'll make up your own mind about whether or not this diet—or any diet—is right for you. If you decide yes, chances are strong you'll make some modifications to make sure the diet meets your needs and allows you the best chance of success.

STRENGTHS: Your greatest asset is that you know your own strengths and weaknesses and plan for them accordingly. You're rarely surprised or caught off guard.

CHALLENGES: Sometimes you can be slow to enter or embrace a new world. Eating PV involves what is usually a radical diet change for most people. You can try to plan and ease into it—for example, giving up wheat one week, oats the next, etc.—but don't expect to see the benefits and results if you're not willing to take a chance and go all in.

MOSTLY B's: THE REALIST

Eyes wide open, this isn't your first rodeo. You better than most understand that changing up your diet is less about drawing a harsh line in the sand and more often about being accepting of the back and forths that come with making any major change or commitment.

STRENGTHS: Grounded, good use of common sense, realistic. With your positive outlook and willingness to not expect perfection 100 percent of the time, you above most have a strong chance of succeeding with the PV diet.

CHALLENGES: Realism can change into cynicism. Also be aware that too much acceptance of "falling off the wagon" can quickly lead to hopping on and off the wagon so much that you end up in circles, going nowhere.

MOSTLY C's: THE COMPETITOR

Like a challenge, do you? You may be deciding to eat PV because you've done the research and are convinced by the science that a diet based on vegetables, smart fat, and high protein makes sense…or someone may have double-dog dared you and now you're in it to win it.

STRENGTHS: An iron will, thriving on challenges, quick to adjust, you enjoy pushing yourself to the limit.

CHALLENGES: Once you're done, you're done. This may translate into your achieving PV perfection for a month and then dropping the whole thing and walking away, looking for the next challenge. Or you may decide from your timed self-experiment that it's something you want to continue, which means you'll need to find a new challenge to distract yourself.

MOSTLY D's: THE DREAMER

Careful there, tiger. While you can't be faulted for your enthusiastic embrace of whatever you put your mind to, there's a danger that you may become disillusioned if and when things don't go exactly according to plan. Cut yourself some slack and allow that just because you're *all in* Monday at 8 a.m., that doesn't mean you're going to feel the same way Thursday night at 7:30 p.m. when you're starving and there's nothing prepared and that pizza delivery is only a phone call away.

STRENGTHS: Enthusiasm, optimism, willingness to jump in and do the work.

CHALLENGES: Enthusiasm quickly turns into discouragement once a challenge or roadblock appears. Beware your tendency toward instant gratification rather than being committed to the long haul and the big picture.

ABOUT THOSE DIETS LISTED IN THE LAST QUESTION...

How many did you check off? There's no right or wrong answer to this (or any of these questions). I just wanted to give you a visual reminder of how many diets you've likely tried out and hopefully remind you that a true diet isn't a "diet" at all.

I really loathe the phrase "healthy eating plan for life" because it's so overused. But eating PV really is about eating whole, healthy foods in abundance. I won't lie. It's not a quick or easy fix. Giving up all the sugar and carbs we've spent decades training our bodies to crave isn't easy. But look where those sugar and carbs have gotten us: bigger and slower with more diabetes, hypertension, and heart disease than ever before.

It's time to take a step back from the "diets" of the world and truly think about what we're putting into our bodies and what results we hope to get from it. That's all.

Chapter 4

A Day in the Life of a Paleo Vegetarian

"Well hey, Dena," you may be saying at this point. "While giving up all grains and beans and most dairy and alienating the better part of my family and friends with a diet they won't understand and in which they'll refuse to participate sure *sounds* swell, I may need just a little more convincing."

I understand. But what you're maybe not seeing is all the benefits that stem from a healthy way of eating. That's why I've put together a quick glimpse of what a day in the life of a Paleo Vegetarian might look like. Take a good look—could this be you?

No Alarm Clock

Awakening based on your body's inner cues is a pleasant way to begin any day. Although I aim to get up at roughly the same time very day, even if I get up 30 minutes earlier or later, I still wake up naturally ten minutes before my alarm goes off. (I still set my alarm because I'm paranoid, but I've probably only had to awaken to it a handful of times in the past year.) Chances are once you're off the sugar/carb cycle, your body will do a better job of self-regulating and you'll be able to wake up on your own versus to the jarring *BZZZ! BZZZ! BZZZ!* of an alarm.

Up and at 'Em

Don't be surprised to find you have a lot more pep in your step in the morning, even if you're not a morning person. PVers wake up feeling refreshed, with no residual bloating or carb coma that accompanies eating a bunch of pasta and rice and bread the night before. We also don't wake up hungry, thanks to the fact that we are now fat-burning and not sugar-burning machines. Yay, us!

First Look in the Mirror

Bye-bye, puffy eyes. And puffy face, for that matter. After two weeks of clean PV eating, even if you haven't lost a pound, you're going to look thinner simply by virtue of not having the puffiness in place that accompanies a high-carb diet. It's still amazing to me when I do eat a flour product, like a bagel, how I almost instantly swell up like a puffer fish. I remember waking up the morning of a marathon race when I'd eaten a prepaid spaghetti with garlic bread dinner the night before. Before I even got out of bed, I thought, "Oh, my." My belly was solid and swollen and my face looked like I'd spent the night crying. It's a treat to look in the mirror each morning on a PV diet and see ourselves for who we really are.

Getting Dressed

Even when I first started running and lost some weight, I still feared getting dressed in the morning. My body had a mind of its own and I never knew what it was planning. Would this be a thin day? A fat day? I kinda-sorta put together that what I ate the day before was influencing my body, but I thought it was more just a simple matter of "I pigged out" that was causing the bloat. Heads up folks—I'm a big eater and I "pig out" every day, only now I do it on healthy PV foods. And thanks to the sugar and carb moderation that implies, I never have to guess what size my body will be each day.

Breakfast

PVers turn things inside, upside, outside down, and this includes the way in which we eat our meals. You're already breaking all the rules so why not push the envelope? My breakfasts these days resemble other people's dinners—maybe some steamed salmon and roasted vegetables with a side of greens. In the winter I cozy up to a steaming bowl of chili or mug of hot soup with a side of asparagus. Every now and again I do the egg/omelet thing, but for some reason, eating "dinner" in the morning always makes me feel full and satisfied until lunch.

Work/Life

Once you're eating a regular PV diet, you're going to feel like someone pumped GO-juice into your veins. You'll feel more energized and alert. If you're eating PV to lose weight, I've also found the diet to be freeing in that I'm not sitting at my desk calculating calories and counting down the minutes until my next "allowed" snack. There is no calorie counting, and if you're hungry, eat something. Just knowing you have the option to eat at any time offers you a huge psychological advantage. We're each of us only equipped with a finite amount of willpower, which gets drained from us each day. Dieters required to use their willpower to follow a strict diet typically find they have limited energy left for home and work projects, and may find themselves procrastinating more than usual. You won't have this problem, since you're not denying yourself food or eating only small portions. Plus, eating healthy fat with each meal (nuts, avocado, coconut oil, egg yolks, etc.) is going to fill you up.

Lunch

I make a big-ass salad the night before and take it to work. And when I say big-ass, I mean behemoth. I start with a base of baby spinach and kale and go from there. Most of my salads have a bevy of roasted vegetables (like peppers, broccoli, brussels sprouts, cauliflower, mushrooms) as well as zucchini and yellow squash, a sliced hard-boiled egg, olives, maybe a small handful of blueberries, and some slivered almonds or pistachios. If I've done a hard workout over lunch, I'll add half of a small baked sweet potato on top. I stuff the salad into a large Tupperware container, but when I pour it onto a plate, I sometimes have to eat it in sections. Otherwise, it doesn't fit. Often what I do is eat half of my big-ass salad for lunch and eat the other part as a snack throughout the day. And before you think, "Eh, salad," let me assure you, this thing rocks. Coworkers see me eating it and start salivating and saying things like, "Oh my God, that looks incredible." Salad power, baby.

Post-Lunch

While the majority of your coworkers stare slack-jawed at their computer screens, fighting off the urge to crawl under their desks for a nap, you, my PV friend, are going to find yourself just as awake and alert at 1 p.m. as you were when you hit the desk at 8 a.m. That's because you haven't sent your insulin levels lunging upward on a grain-based sugar high only to have them plummet and leave you feeling tired, drained, and—yes—hungry. Should you annoy coworkers with your "I'm so awake and happy and you're not" buoyancy? I say you only live once so sure, why not?

Eat When You're Hungry

It's almost gospel diet advice that in order to lose weight, you need to eat five or six small meals throughout the day. The rationale is that doing so keeps your blood sugars level. As PV eaters, we know that if we avoid foods that spike the levels in the first place, there's no need to eat five or six times a day to level them out. *Can* you eat that many meals a day? So long as you stick to PV-approved foods, sure. But I challenge you instead to start listening to your body. Most of us have been dieting for so long that the concept of eating when our body tells us it's hungry is a foreign concept. Instead, we eat according to the clock, spacing our little meals out like soldiers on a battlefield in the fight against fat.

Give it a shot. Eat only when you're hungry. If you're not hungry until 10:52 a.m., then eat breakfast at 10:52 a.m. If you're not hungry after that until 7:39 p.m., then eat at 7:39 p.m. Or if you find yourself hungry again at 11:31 a.m., eat at 11:31 a.m.

The fact is that most of us have no idea what real hunger feels like. I'm not saying that you should wait until you go into a swoon before eating, but I am suggesting that you make sure you're eating based on hunger and not external clues. For example, we see our coworkers packing up their purse to head out to lunch or we smell the garlicky aroma of last night's pasta dinner being heated up in the company microwave and we think, "Time to eat," without ever really questioning if we're hungry.

To reengage with your body I suggest you do the *other* piece of diet gospel advice and keep a journal. Just for a short while until you get into the groove of things. More important than tracking food (which I believe is helpful, but which, if I'm being honest, bores me to tears and I never last longer than three days) is tracking *why* you're eating. Looking over my past food journals I find the same reasons appearing over and over again:

- Joined coworkers for lunch
- Bored
- Ate because I knew I wouldn't have a chance to eat later and didn't want to risk getting hungry
- Stressed about work
- Bored
- Wasn't hungry for dinner but ate anyway knowing I have a big workout in the morning
- Procrastinating on project—ate my lunch and snacks early instead
- Bored
- Stressed and bored
- Had dinner plans with friends; not really hungry but ate a full meal
- Wanted something to go with my coffee
- Lunchtime
- Bored, bored, bored

See a theme? You can even hear it in the way people talk to each other. "Do you want to eat now or later?" "Whenever. I'm not starving but I can always eat."

It takes practice, but learning to pause before you push in that first mouthful to ask yourself "Why am I eating this?" will save you unwanted pounds—so long as you have the presence of mind to set the fork down if the answer isn't "Because I'm hungry!"

Exercise

I'm going to share an insight with you that took me years to learn and embrace. Lean in, because this is important. Ready? Here it is: You don't need to eat before a workout. Seriously. You'll have plenty of energy on an empty stomach.

Perhaps it's the runner in me, but I had it ingrained in my psyche that in order to perform—or even get through—a hard workout, I better damn well carb up in advance. Otherwise, I would run out of energy and then where would I be? So I spent years and years and *years* loading up on bagels and apples and bananas and peanut butter in the early mornings before a workout. And for almost a decade it was a given that Friday was pasta night at our house, given that I had a long run the next day. Didn't matter if my "long" run was 5 miles or 25 miles, I ate pasta and breadsticks like a starved Italian.

It was only after I started eating Paleo and reading about it that I found the courage to try working out without a stomach full of bread or fruit. The result? Bing! My workouts didn't suffer. At all. Let me qualify this and say this is for workouts that last under an hour. If you're going to be doing a 90-minute or two-hour run, you'll still find it helpful to eat something beforehand (more on this later). But on weekdays when most of us hit the gym at lunch or before work for a 50-minute spin class or 30 minutes of weight training, you can work out on an empty stomach. In fact, studies show that what's called "fasted training" can actually improve performance. The key, it turns out, isn't eating before you work out. It's eating after to help aid muscle recovery. (More on this later, too.)

All of this is to say that if you are exercising, it's okay to go to the gym first thing in the morning or before lunch or dinner without eating. Grab a small handful of nuts if you feel like you need something, but give working out on an empty stomach a try and see if you don't pump those weights a little harder, row a little faster, or take an extra lap around the track.

Dinner

Mmmm…so much Paleo Vegetarian goodness from which to choose! If you like to cook, now is the time to experiment. However, if cooking isn't your thing, there's nothing wrong with keeping things simple and eating the same meals over and over again. Along with my "dinner for breakfast" bit, one of my favorite things to do is to swap it out and eat breakfast at night. At least three times a week, I'll make a big veggie omelet or a simple plate of scrambled eggs and greens for dinner. Fills me up and I'm in and out of the kitchen in less than ten minutes. Give it a try.

Relaxing

On diets in the past, so much of my time was spent tied up thinking about my diet and what I could and couldn't eat and when I could eat it, that I forgot to enjoy life. I hope you won't let that happen on a PV diet. Family, friends, pets, and hobbies make a life. Food is a distant second.

PV is more than a way of eating. It's closer to a mindset and a lifestyle, one in which you choose to be healthy, understanding that health is a multifaceted experience and the food we eat is only a small part of that. Now that you're no longer feeling sluggish or manic from a diet heavy in carbs and sugar, you'll have extra energy. So do what makes you happy. Go for a walk, read a book, snuggle with the kids on the couch for a movie, make over the spare bedroom, clean out the garage, paint a picture, write a book.

I have no scientific evidence to back this claim up, but speaking from personal experience I can tell you that when I feel in charge of my diet, I feel in charge of my life. I'm more motivated to plow through a to-do list or meet up with friends or tackle a project. Part of it is, I'm sure, the sustained energy that comes from clean eating. An equal or larger part, however, is mental. When I used to fail on diets, I felt like I was failing in life. So if I ate over calorie count—which I always did because I was *hungry*—I felt like I hadn't just blown my diet, but the whole day. Maybe the whole week.

You'll never feel like that on PV. If you slip one day, or one meal, you've got the 80/20 principle, so it will be okay. And this isn't a diet of denial. You may get a little bored eating PV, but you should never be hungry. If you are, eat. What other diet tells you that?

Sweet Dreams

Adequate sleep is underrated as the foundational tool for weight loss. PVers who are serious about weight loss get plenty of sleep. Why the extra shut eye? Because a lack of sleep has been shown over and over again to cause an increase in hunger, leading to weight gain.

Why would lack of sleep make us hungry? Wouldn't the extra time spent awake actually help us burn more calories?

Aw, that's cute. You're so tired you're actually hallucinating.

Nope, it doesn't work that way. Here's how it does: When you skimp on the sleep, you're stressing your body. To fight the stress, your body produces the stress hormone cortisol. Cortisol is there to rev up your metabolism and give you energy, helping you through stressful periods. But cortisol also releases insulin, giving you that "fight-or-flight" kick in the pants that revs up your appetite for starchy, sugary, high-carbohydrate foods. So, less sleep equals more insulin, which equals more craving for carbs and sugar. More cravings for carbs and sugar equals hunger pangs. Hunger pangs typically lead to overeating sugary, high-carbohydrate foods, which leads to weight gain.

Take away: Get your shut eye. And plenty of it. What's plenty? At least seven hours a night. A 2004 study reported on WebMD found that getting less than six hours of sleep a night made people 30 percent more likely to become obese when compared to people who were logging seven to nine hours a night.

Especially when it comes to weight loss, getting enough sleep isn't just a luxury, it's a necessity. Remember that.

Chapter 5

Moving into the Right Mindset

Abundance versus Deprivation

Here's the thing. Starting out, maintaining a Paleo Vegetarian diet will feel hard. I know when I first made the commitment to eat PV, I went through my pantry, refrigerator, and freezer and ruthlessly eliminated anything that didn't fit with the Paleo diet. Out went the bulk bags of dried pinto and black beans! Out went the Bob's Red Mill boxes of quinoa, amaranth, barley, and couscous! Out went $200 worth of soy-based meatballs, deli meat, veggie patties, and my beloved soy sausage crumbles. When the comeuppance was over and I had carried a bulging trash bag to the curb,[10] I remember returning to my kitchen and staring into the recesses of my pantry, barren now except for some sweet potatoes and a can of black olives that had been nesting there for the better part of a year and thinking, "What am I going to *eat?*"

---

10 Or delight a vegetarian friend or neighbor with your bounty of no-no foods for you. Your loss, their gain. (Probably literally. Oooh—shouldn't have gone there.)

You've Been Here Before

Here's the good news. As practicing vegetarians, most of us have been here before and come out on the other side. When you began your vegetarian journey, you likely experienced the sense of helplessness that accompanies making any decision to radically alter a diet. When you did the cupboard stripping that comes with committing to a vegetarian lifestyle and forced yourself to dispose of the cans of StarKist, the packets of bacon, the deli-wrapped hamburger meat, and the small, seemingly innocent packs of Jell-O (remember when you found out *Jell-O* wasn't vegetarian? *Mind. Blowing.*), you too looked deep into the fridge and the depth of your soul and thought, "Holy crap! There is *nothing* here I can eat!"

And Yet You Thrived

You learned better. You discovered there was an endless variety of foods to eat as a vegetarian, and yes, I promise you, there is an endless variety of foods and meal combinations to be discovered as a Paleo Vegetarian. Assuming you ate reasonably healthy as a vegetarian, your kitchen cupboards aren't going to look dramatically different as a Paleo Vegetarian. There will be an abundance of vegetables, particularly those of the big, leafy green variety. Beets, yams, sweet potatoes, squash, peppers, tomatoes, onions, eggplant, brussels sprouts, avocados, nuts… these will be the staples of your new diet.

My advice is to be patient. It took months before the vegetarian lifestyle began to resonate with me and cooking a batch of quinoa with leafy greens for a main meal felt natural and filling. It will be the same with Paleo Vegetarianism. At first, the meals may feel lacking or incomplete without grains as a foundation upon which you build your menu. Soon, however, forgoing grains will feel as natural and easy as skipping a steak or pork chop feels to you now.

The Mad Scientist

Choosing the foods with which you nourish your body becomes a combined act of science and love. I still remember the first day I looked at a doughnut and had no desire to eat it simply because I was mentally calculating the fat and sugar and damage it would do. Instead of thinking, "I wish…" I thought, "No way." I literally wasn't even tempted. That won't always be the case, but as your mind changes around food and you start paying attention to what you eat and how your body responds to different foods and different food combinations, you may be surprised to find some of your hardcore temptations no longer hold sway over you. And that, my friends, is a fine day indeed.

Food Is Just Food

Getting into the right mindset often requires taking a step back and reviewing the bigger picture. What makes you happy? Do you have people who love you and who you show love in return? Do you have a job that—even if you don't love it—affords you a place to live, a means of transportation, cable, a cell phone, and the ability to provide for your family? Does your dog think you're the bomb? Does your cat at least tolerate you?

These are all powerful, wonderful things that 99 percent of the world would love to have and for which they would be more than willing to trade away their ideal weight. I don't know you personally, but I'm guessing that if you have the time and inclination to read a book on Paleo Vegetarianism, things are going well for you in life. This doesn't imply any level of being shallow. It simply means that there is, as Maslow pointed out, a hierarchy of needs humans follow. Most of us, and I certainly lump myself into this group, can become so focused on what we don't have or what we want that we forget to take into account all the "ordinary" miracles that fill our day. Things like having enough money to put gas in our car or tucking our kids in at night or having a selection of fresh produce at our fingertips every time we go to the store.

Reminding yourself of everything that is going right in your life is actually an excellent diet strategy. Doing this demonstrates to you all the success you've already experienced in other aspects of your life and is a reminder that there's no reason you can't experience the same success in your eating and health habits as well.

Overcoming Roadblocks and Challenges

Your beliefs become your thoughts,
Your thoughts become your words,
Your words become your actions,
Your actions become your habits,
Your habits become your values,
Your values become your destiny.

—*Mahatma Gandhi*

Think happy thoughts.

—*Peter Pan*

Too often, we judge ourselves solely on our actions. Did we eat the cookie or let it go? Did we stop eating when we were full or did we insist on cleaning our plate until we were stuffed? Did we drink enough water, get enough sleep, eat something green with every meal?

Actions, actions, actions. The actions we choose are the success or failure of our diets. But what drives us to pursue one course of action over another?

TIP #1: HOW YOU THINK ABOUT FOOD CAN HELP YOU EAT BETTER

When I was a freelance writer, I spent the better part of my days in local coffeehouses, writing. One day soon after I'd adopted the Paleo Vegetarian lifestyle, the apron-clad store owner of our local coffeehouse approached me. He waved a tray of fresh-from-the-oven, gooey, sugar-laden chocolate-chip cookies in front of my nose.

"Have one," he said. "On the house."

(Let me pause here to mention that I *love* chocolate-chip cookies. All kinds—homemade, out of the box, stale, Keebler-elf imprinted... they are all delicious to me.)

I took a deep breath, trying not to inhale heavenly cookie scent. "Thank you," I said. "I appreciate it, but I'm going to have to pass. I'm trying not to eat grains."

Good for me! Right? Well, sort of.

Can you spot the misstep? Read over what I said. See it now? The potential downfall of my diet is right there in the word "trying."

When you tell others you're "trying" not to eat grains or you're "trying" to give up dairy or you're "hoping" to convert to Paleo Vegetarianism, what you're really doing is telling them—and yourself—that eating this way isn't something you've fully committed to.

"Trying" implies wiggle room. "Trying" leaves the door open for "Maybe I'll do better tomorrow." Look at your choice to be a vegetarian. Generally speaking, you don't "try" to not eat meat. You. Don't. Eat. Meat. Period. It's simply who you are.

So what should my response (and your response) to someone offering me (you) a cookie have been? Something more along the lines of, "Thank you, that's generous of you to offer and I'm sorry to say no, but I don't eat grains."

> When you say to others "I'm trying not to eat grains," or "I'm trying to eat Paleo Vegetarian," what you're really doing is telling them—and yourself—that this is a path to which you have not yet fully committed.

It's polite but definitive. It also shuts the door on discussion. With "I'm trying not to," you leave yourself open to people encouraging you to splurge "just this one time." And why not? You've just told them you're only "trying," so obviously there are times when you're allowing yourself to fall off the no-grain wagon. However, notice the difference when you hear someone (like you!) state that they don't eat grains, period. There's nowhere for the discussion to go when your response to every "just this one time" encouragement is a firm, "Thank you, but I don't eat grains."

You do need to watch your thoughts as they become your words, and watch your words as they become your actions. However, it's possible to reverse engineer this situation. Every time you state aloud that you don't eat grains or that you follow a Paleo Vegetarian diet—even if you don't yet fully trust yourself to do so— you're further embedding that truth in your psyche. And sooner than you think, the true belief will take hold and passing up that cookie becomes not so much a battle of willpower as it's simply who you are.

TIP #2: NOW THAT YOU'RE THINKING ABOUT FOOD IN A BETTER WAY, QUIT THINKING ABOUT IT SO MUCH

Do we ever stop obsessing about food? If I had a dime for every minute spent thinking, dreaming, worrying, obsessing, planning, or berating myself over my food choices, I'd be rich enough that I could move to my own private island far away from prying eyes and eat my fill of whatever food I want.

I don't know many of us out there who don't obsess about food, at least to some degree, and that includes people who say they have no interest in eating healthier. Start paying attention to how people talk about food and you'll hear it. It's the coworker sighing, "I really shouldn't," as she bites into a sugary cupcake brought in to celebrate the boss's birthday. It's in the hesitation of the woman perusing the dinner menu, debating ordering what she *wants* versus what she thinks she *should* order. A focus on food is even found in the "I don't care what I eat" braggart who returns to the table with a towering plate of fried food from the all-you-can-eat buffet and proudly declares, "This is living!" before digging in. It's the people standing in line at Wendy's and McDonald's who let their gaze linger on the burgers and fries before ordering the grilled chicken salad (or not). It's the health nut who obsessively tracks every morsel of healthy food that goes into his lean, sculpted body.

But what is all this obsession about food gaining us? As far as I can tell, it's bringing most of us a lot of guilt. And guilt, for as much as we drag it around with us, is a useless emotion. Useless, but dangerous.

When we inflict dietary guilt on ourselves, we're doing so in the belief and hope that "punishing" ourselves this way will lead to wiser choices the next go-round. In fact, choosing to experience guilt over a dietary lapse usually leads to more lapses. One study[11] showed that when we feel guilty we *literally* feel heavier. The same study showed that guilt—and the feeling of weight that

---

11 http://www.plosone.org/article/info%3Adoi%2F10.1371%2Fjournal.
    pone.0069546

accompanies it—made exercising feel harder. Yikes! Exercising made *harder*? Who needs that?

Bottom line: While I'm not advocating a moral free-for-all, use common sense when it comes to your diet. You're not going to make yourself healthier by feeling bad about yourself. So you ate a bagel. Let it go and move on.[12]

TIP #3: THINK THOUGHTS OF GRATITUDE

I'm not talking about food here. Think thoughts of gratitude about your life. Go as big picture or as granular as you like. Studies show that feelings of gratitude breed happiness and well-being. If you're the writerly type, keep a journal. Write down three things each morning or each night for which you're grateful. Maybe it's the laugh of your child or the waking up to the hot, stinky breath of your dog (who is *so* happy that you're finally awake!). If you don't like to write, make a pact with your partner (or your dog) to say aloud each morning three things for which you're grateful or that make you happy.

Since it's the little details of life that tend to bog me down, I find my spirits lifted when I pull back and look at the big picture. Okay, so there are ants in my bathroom and my car is making a weird noise. My gratitude list this week included enjoying a coffee with a friend, completing a hard long run at my goal pace, seeing a cardinal outside my window, and getting a free perfume sample in the mail. I also like to remind myself that I have a job, food in my fridge, a healthy body and mind, and a life filled with friends, freedom, and way too much cat hair.

---

12 One more reason to let it go: orthorexia nervosa, the clinically defined obsession with healthy eating. Food should be only one aspect of a full, healthy life. If you find every moment of your life filled with thoughts of what you can eat, when can you eat it, and how "good or bad" it is for you, be aware you're heading down a dangerous—and unhealthy—path of obsession.

The goal here is to cultivate feelings of abundance in every area of your life. Feeling gratitude about life will make it easier to stick to your dietary goals.

TIP #4: BE KIND TO YOURSELF

How's your internal dialogue? Would you talk to another person the way you talk to yourself? Most of us would dial it back a notch. You are your own worst critic, but with a little conscious effort, you can also be your biggest fan.

When I ran a job-search program at a women's center for displaced homemakers, I was appalled at the self-criticism and negativity I heard coming from program participants. Several of the women were staying in dead-end jobs or relationships because they felt they had no choice. I asked one of the women who was in a dangerous relationship, what if it was her daughter in this relationship? Would she want her to stay?

"Of course not!" said the woman.

"Why?" I asked.

"Because she deserves better. I want her to be happy."

"So why would you want any less for yourself?"

For some reason, many of us can see the potential in others but have a hard time seeing the same in ourselves. Start paying attention to how you talk to yourself, around both food and life in general. If you find yourself being overly critical, stop and ask if you would be so hard on someone else—your son, your daughter, your partner, a parent, a friend. Remind yourself you're worthy of the same love and support you so willingly bestow upon others.

TIP #5: IT'S YOUR DIET—QUIT ANNOYING OTHERS WITH IT

I say this as a friend. Please, please, please shut up already about your food choices. As a woman who has come perilously close to alienating both friends and family with my enthusiastic (some might say "annoyingly obsessive") embrace of healthy eating, I know that of which I speak. It's natural to want to share your knowledge with others, especially when you see how PV eating starts to unlock the secrets of weight loss, sustained energy, glowing skin, and lack of sugar cravings. All I can say is, wait for people to come to you. No one wants to be told what they're eating is terrible for them. (I'm embarrassed to admit that I used to be—and okay, sometimes still am—that girl who stands in the middle of the chip aisle at the grocery store and loudly proclaims, "I cannot believe people actually eat this crap!") Besides, don't you think they already know that the candy bar is bad for them?

Another reason not to proselytize is because people will come to you, wanting to know your secret, once they see you dropping weight and looking healthy and energized. If they do ask what your secret is, then that's the time to share. Even then, a little information goes a long way. There's no need to load them up with every detail of a PV diet.[13] A Paleo and/or vegetarian diet is more than most people can get their minds around. Tie the two together and you're in danger of short-circuiting someone's brain. Have an elevator speech handy on what a PV diet, is but limit your spiel to one or two main points you think may help them, such as, "I found eliminating grains has really spurred my weight loss."

---

13 Unless you want to contribute to my retirement fund and buy them a copy of this book in which case, yes, by all means, load them up with info!

Explaining Your Choice to Others (Because They'll Ask!)

Whether you're pescatarian, lacto-vegetarian, vegan, macrobiotic, or full-on Paleo, people are going to ask you about your food choices. And they're not just going to ask, they're going to judge. How many of us still deal with "You don't eat *meat*? Well, that's just stupid. You can't be getting enough protein," accompanied by the not-so-subtle dismissive sniff. (Thanks, Mom.)

We've all been through this particular drama before with our decision to be vegetarians. When the office brings in pizza for lunch and your coworkers loudly announce that one is a *plain cheese for Dena because she doesn't eat meat* or when you show up for dinner at a friend's house, casserole pot in hand because you didn't want her to go to the extra trouble of cooking a special vegan dish just for you, these and other times are when the spotlight shines on you as people turn to you and say, "Tell me again why you don't eat meat?"

Now add in the Paleo aspect of not eating grains, dairy, soy, or rice, and trust me, your friends and family are going to lose their freaking minds.

While there's no law that says you have to explain your choice to others, most of us feel obligated to offer some sort of reply. A simple shrug and smile might be enough to end the conversation. Or you may feel the need to give an ethics lesson on animal cruelty and why your choice to not eat meat is based on moral standings. I think it was sometime around my third year as a vegetarian that I noticed I was no longer being asked to parties, evidence suggesting that the other guests munching on beef sliders and chicken wings didn't appreciate my unprovoked tirades about the different ways chickens and cows are tortured so we could be the beneficiaries of cheap meat.

Just remember that you don't have to defend yourself or your dietary choices. You can, but ask yourself what you're hoping to gain before you enter an all-out war with someone over the evils of grains. Do you think by explaining your choices you'll turn them on to your way of eating? It's not likely to happen. Do you want to educate them? Most people will tune out a lecture.

Depending on whom I'm dealing with and what I know of them, I carry a few simple back-pocket strategies that I pull out as needed.

EXAMINE THE EXAMINER

For the person I don't know well who starts a conversation with something along the lines of, "Oh God, you're one of those crazy Paleo people," I offer up something along the lines of, "Uh-oh, sounds like you're not a fan. What part is it about the Paleo diet that you don't agree with?" Chances are these people know nothing about Paleo. All they know is that it's some new "diet craze." And they'll be forced to stand there in front of you and admit that they know very little about the intricacies of the diet. And this, friends, I won't lie, is very, very satisfying to hear them admit.

TALK ABOUT WHAT YOU DO EAT INSTEAD OF WHAT YOU DON'T

Here's a little party trick I learned as a vegetarian that can also serve you well as a Paleo Vegetarian. I would ask the person standing before me, explaining to me how limited my diet is because I don't eat meat, what he or she had for dinner last night. Most people cook fairly boring, so the answer was usually "spaghetti," "burgers," or "We ate out."

"Okay," I'd say. "Here's what I had. Last night I sat down to a chilled eggplant and sun-dried tomato salad followed by a pumpkin squash soup, and a shiitake and bok choy sauté with roasted julienned vegetables entrée sprinkled with a sesame seed dressing. For dessert I had coffee with heavy whipping cream and dark chocolate–covered walnuts and berries."

Now, the trick to this is to memorize a good meal and have it ready to go. You may know that last night you just noshed on almond butter and a banana, but they don't know that and the point is you *could* have had that delicious meal and will on most nights. Shameless? Maybe. But the fact is everyone appreciates a good meal description (just ask the Food Network), and once people realize you're not nibbling on nuts and berries you foraged yourself for every meal, they're usually a little more willing to listen.

PULL OUT THE STATS

A little knowledge goes a long way. For people who are determined to get in your face about your diet—and if you decide you want to get in their face back—nothing is more powerful than having facts at hand. When I was a vegetarian, I used to quote from *The China Study* about cancer and mortality rates and how long meat stayed in a person's digestive tract. For Paleo Vegetarian, the main question you'll be asked is, "What's wrong with bread?" Know your stuff and have an answer ready to go.

STEER AWAY FROM FEATURES AND TALK ABOUT BENEFITS

I work in marketing, and a golden rule is that you're never selling a product, you're selling the experience of how that product makes you feel. Take do-it-yourself, at-home hair-coloring kits, i.e., Ms. Clairol. They're not selling darker roots. They're selling looking younger and feeling confident and in control.

Similarly, when you talk about your diet and eating choices, don't focus on features, like what you do and do not eat. Talk up the benefits. So a feature of a Paleo Vegetarian diet is that you don't eat grains. Not much fun to talk about. But a *benefit* of the diet is that you have more energy, your skin looks great, and your stomach is flat because it's no longer bloated from all the gluten.

Whether it's warding off disease, having more energy, or simply feeling on top of and in control of your life both mentally and physically, talk up the PV benefits that mean the most to you. Most people will have a hard time arguing with these.

This isn't to imply that eating PV means you're about to be attacked 24/7. Recognize most questioning for what it is—people are curious as to what you're doing and your reasons for doing it. Some of them, like family members (hi, Mom), will be worried you're jumping on a fad diet and wrecking your health with those "weird diet ideas." Understand that while they might not always phrase it exactly right, most people who care about you aren't attacking—they simply want to make sure you're doing what's best for you and your health.

And don't discount the fact that others will be asking what you're doing because they've seen a difference in you and want a part of the magic elixir that brought you there. When you're able to start someone else on a journey to health not by lecturing or cajoling but through being a living example of the results they want in their life, you're going to feel very, very good about yourself and the choices you've made.

Chapter 6

Paleo Vegetarian Diet 101

Opposite Ends of the Spectrum: Carb Coma versus Low-Carb Flu

The first time I ever heard reference to a "carb coma" was while watching *The Biggest Loser* TV show. The contestants had been given the challenge to eat a smorgasbord of their favorite sugary, starchy, dairy, and gluten-laden foods, all in the hopes of earning the golden ticket—a 2-pound advantage at weigh-in. Half the contestants dove in, eating candy bars, hot dogs, pizza, pasta, cookies, doughnuts, and more. I have no idea who won, but what I do remember are the reactions of trainers Bob Harper and Jillian Michaels once the feeding frenzy ended. The trainers entered the room where the contestants were scattered glassy-eyed and bloated. I recall watching Bob Harper, disgusted with the group, point to a contestant and saying something along the lines of, "Tara is sitting over there in such a carb coma she can barely move."

And the thing was, even through the TV, I could see what he was talking about. The contestants were sitting there numb, glassy-eyed, and just *dull* looking. It was a noticeable, visual difference from the contestants around them who'd chosen not to partake in the game. Obviously pounds of weight hadn't instantly appeared on the contestants but just looking at them, you could tell they felt heavier.

Carb comas are real and I'm willing to bet you've experienced them, and much more frequently than you may realize.

"CARB COMA" DEFINED

The fancy name for a carb coma is "postprandial somnolence." And what is that, exactly? An overly simplified definition is that it's drowsiness related to glucose entering the bloodstream due to the type of food that's just been consumed.

Why do these attacks of drowsiness occur? Contrary to what we've been told, carbohydrates in and of themselves are not the enemy. Our bodies and minds need carbohydrates for energy. But all carbs are not created equal. Junk food as well as many of the carbohydrates that are part of a "healthy" diet (think whole-grain bagel with peanut butter or fruit-on-the-bottom yogurt) more quickly converts to sugar in the bloodstream. This in turn produces a rise of insulin as your body struggles to maintain normal blood sugar levels and move the "toxic" glucose out. It does this in one of two ways. First, it shoves the extra sugar into muscles. But we only have limited storage space there so guess what? All the excess glucose gets converted to fat. Yippee.

Next is the roller-coaster ride. You've felt that swift, jittery, sometimes nauseous feeling that comes with either eating too much food or even just eating small amounts of certain foods such as sweets? As insulin floods your system to drive down blood sugar levels, your body is thrown into a state of chaos, often referred to as a sugar rush. However, what goes up must come down. As the insulin does its job and pushes the glucose out of your bloodstream and into your fat cells, your blood sugar levels drop, causing you to feel thick, heavy, and lethargic. Sound familiar? Congratulations. The sugar crash has set in.

Unfortunately, this merry-go-round of up and down is a daily occurrence for millions of Americans who take it for granted they will feel dazed and sleepy upon returning to the office after lunch. Sugar is the primary culprit. But this pattern (often repeated at breakfast, lunch, dinner, and with snacks) takes a toll on the body, creating a vicious cycle of inflammation that stresses the body to the core, each and every day.

Is it worth it? Along with the feelings of drowsiness and lethargy also come the feelings of helplessness and self-loathing. We hate that we feel bloated and out of control. We swear we'll never overeat like that again. Or we promise we'll confine ourselves to a mere taste of the sugary foods that cause the peaks and valleys. And we mean it. Until the next time rolls around…

LOW-CARB FLU: TRANSITIONING FROM A HIGH-CARB DIET

Let's jump to the opposite end of the spectrum. Obviously carb comas are bad news, both in terms of what they do to the body and how they make you feel. The good news is that eating Paleo Vegetarian means you will end, once and for all, the cycle of sugar highs and lows and the doldrums that accompany that way of eating. Let's face it; it's pretty challenging to drag yourself into a carb coma on a diet that consists primarily of vegetables.

However, if your diet has previously been heavy in carbs—and most every vegetarian's diet is—you may experience a transition period that will leave you feeling, well, crappy.

The carb flu or low-carb flu refers to a set of symptoms that occur as the body detoxes from its carb-laden state. (Another way to think of it is the transition period as your body moves from being sugar burning to fat burning.) Not everyone experiences carb flu and there seems to be no rhyme or reason for who does and who doesn't. But if, as you begin your PV journey, you feel any or all of the symptoms below, recognize that you're not sick, you're not dying, and this diet isn't "terrible because of how it makes me feel." Feeling "meh" for a short time actually means you're on the way to feeling much better each and every day for the rest of your life.

THE DOCTOR IS IN

You may be experiencing a version of low-carb flu if, after starting to eat PV, you experience:

- Aches and shakiness

- Headaches

- Mental fog or fuzziness (forgetting things)

- Constant tiredness/fatigue

- Mood swings

- Difficulty completing workouts

These symptoms may last anywhere from a few days to a few weeks. Wait—a few *weeks*? Yup. Which is why it's important you have a heads-up that it may be coming. Otherwise, if you're feeling constantly drained of energy, with a low-grade headache and achy joints, you're going to jump to the logical-seeming (yet incorrect) conclusion that this diet is horrible for you and your health.

If you do get hit with the low-carb flu, there are some things you can try to alleviate the symptoms. These include:

- Staying hydrated
- Getting at least seven to eight hours of sleep each night
- Eating more healthy fats such as avocados, olive/coconut oils, real butter or ghee, whole eggs, nuts
- Eating a little protein and fat before a workout
- Reducing the intensity of your workouts until the symptoms pass, especially if you're doing high-intensity workouts that last over an hour

Remember, low-carb flu is simply your body transitioning from using unhealthy glucose carbs to the more ideal situation of creating glucose from healthy fats and proteins. The symptoms will pass and you'll not only return to normal, you'll return to a state of amped-up, feeling *better* than normal that will make you wonder how you ever used to get through your day in your zombielike carb-coma state.

Don't Fear the Fat

I love the look of shock on people's faces when I explain to them that I eat a high-fat diet. We, all of us, have been brainwashed for so long to think "low-fat" that we don't even question the reasoning behind it any longer. But the SnackWells era of "OMG—there is *no fat* in these cookies! Here, let's split a box" made us all—you guessed it—fat.

Is it true you can lose weight on a high-fat diet? Yes, it is. And do you want to know the two best things about eating fat?

1. Fat tastes REALLY good.
2. Fat fills you up.

I know, right? Like Halloween and Christmas all rolled into one. Naturally, not all fat is created equal. While I would love to tell you that the fat found in a Reese's Peanut Butter Cups is the good healthy kind, um, no. Unfortunately, I can't do it. (But rest assured if that ever happens, I will phone you immediately.)

There are, however, a number of phenomenally healthy fats out there in which you may feel free to indulge. And—this is the fun part—you finally get a leg up on all your friends and family who have mocked, questioned, or challenged your diet. What, Cousin Jessica, you're forgoing butter on your dinner roll because it's fattening? Huh. Well, I'm just going to drown my vegetables in some real butter[14] and say, "Mmmmmm…." in front of you while I eat them. (Yeah, Jessica and I have issues.)

Fats will be a key part in your dieting success. Take a deep breath and read that again. Don't just gloss over the words. Embrace them. **Fats help you lose weight.** This is important. I'm serious about the brainwashing. We are a country that fears fat. But if you're going to make the PV diet work for you, you need to overcome any mental block you have to eating fat. It really is the key to filling you up and helping you crave less food, thereby assisting in long-term weight loss.

So come, join me on a tour of what I like to call the fun and fantastic world of fats.

FAT AT A GLANCE

There's a world of research available on fats—saturated versus unsaturated and the role of cholesterol and the family of omegas. Google search "Paleo fats" and you'll find long diatribes with complicated-looking equations and chemical compounds. We're not going into all that here. But I will give you a quick insight into

---

14 If you're a pescatarian Paleo Vegetarian, it's fun to do this with lobster. While everyone else at the table is delicately dipping their crustacean into butter, moaning about calories, you can dunk away without a care, a big smile on your lobster-eating face.

the role fat plays in the PV world and why the Paleo view on fat differs so radically from that of conventional medical wisdom.

There are three primary categories of fatty acids: saturated fats, monounsaturated fats, and polyunsaturated fats. Let's focus on saturated fat. Why? Because it's gotten such a bad rap. People tend to lump cholesterol and saturated fat into one great big "no-no" category. "Death by cholesterol! Heart-clogging disease!" These are but a few of the rallying cries of conventional wisdom against eating saturated fats. So why do Paleoists embrace them?

Saturated fats are essential to body function. Intake of saturated fats plays a key role in brain function and cardiovascular benefits and help with everything from calcium absorption for strong bones to boosting our immune systems. In fact, new studies indicate that heart disease and obesity is caused not by saturated fats (like eggs, red meat, butter, cheese) but by "healthy" unsaturated foods like corn and vegetable oils. Saturated fats taste good and fill you up. They're a "yes" on a Paleo-based diet.

Next is monounsaturated fats. The Paleo take on these fats is that they are good for you so long as they aren't heated, as this causes a breakdown of free radicals. (Insert complicated chemical-chain graphic here...*yawn.*) Monounsaturated fats lower blood cholesterol concentrations and are found in foods like olive oil, nuts, and avocados.

Now for the bad boys, the polyunsaturated fats (cue scary music). For once, conventional wisdom has it right. These fats are not good for you, as our bodies can't metabolize them. You'll find most polyunsaturated fats hiding behind names like "hydrogenated" or "partially hydrogenated" on the ingredient list. Often these fats are used to give foods a long shelf life.

And finally, trans fat. No section on fats would be complete without mention of trans fats. Found in most any form of junk food and frequently listed as "partially hydrogenated" on the ingredients list, trans fats are unhealthy and throw the body into a tailspin. They're also a common cause behind weight gain. Avoid, avoid, avoid!

THE OMEGA FAMILY

Omega-3s and omega-6s are both necessary for our health. However, the standard American diet is heavy in omega-6s and generally lacking in omega-3s. What foods contain omega-3s? Wild-caught fish, eggs, and nuts are the standout stars; although lower in concentration, dark green vegetables like broccoli and spinach also contain amounts of these healthy fats. Flax seeds and walnuts are wonderful, and even though not Paleo (but possibly included in a modified PV diet), beans contain good amounts of omega-3s as well. That's your overview. Now let's dig into some of the actual ingredients you can and should be using in your PV diet.

WHAT PV FATS SHOULD I BE EATING?

To say that Paleo folks love their fats is like saying that race car drivers like to occasionally step on the gas. Uh, *yeah they do.* As Paleo Vegetarians, we adopt the same fat-loving mindset of pure Paleoists, if not the exact same set of fats. True Paleo relies heavily on animal fats. Beef lard, bacon drippings, poultry fat, tallow, duck fat…Paleo recipe websites are literally dripping in animal fat.

That's not our bag. So what fats as Paleo Vegetarians can and should we be eating?

Butter

Or as I like to call it, "butt-ahhh." When it comes to livening up foods, the saying "Everything's better with butter" isn't just a tagline, it's a mantra. Butter has a low smoke point, so it's not great for high-temperature cooking, but there aren't many foods I can think of that won't benefit from a little butter poured over them, especially fish and fresh veggies. Ideally you want your butter to come from a grass-fed cow as it will contain more CLAs, or conjugated linoleic acids. Even if the term sounds ominous, CLAs are our friends. Studies are showing CLAs help reduce body fat, increase muscle strength, and help with endurance workouts.

Ghee

Ghee is clarified butter, meaning butter with all of the milk solids removed. In other words, it's pure fat. Or in other, other words, pure heaven. It has a much higher smoke point than butter, making it ideal for sautés. It also has a slightly nuttier flavor than butter, which is really, really good when preparing eggs and veggies. Did I already use the word "heaven"? I did. Well, ghee deserves a double dose: It's heavenly.

Olive Oil

Olive oil is also 100 percent fat. (Notice a trend here?) Aside from being mostly monounsaturated healthy fat, olive oil also serves up healthy doses of vitamins E and K. It has a low smoke point and may not be ideal for cooking, but it's perfect for cold dressings or as a healthy drizzle on top of your meals. Go for extra-virgin olive oil for higher quality and a stronger flavor.

Coconut Oil

Say hello to your new best friend. Coconut anything is often hailed as king in the Paleo world, and you'll find coconut used in a lot of recipes, especially Paleo desserts, where coconut flour reigns supreme. As a fat, however, coconut oil has a lot going for it. It's solid at room temperature due to the fact that it's mostly saturated fat. *Gasp.* Saturated fat? But…but…isn't that the bad stuff?

Yes, if it's found in a Taco Bell burrito. No, if it's found in coconut oil. What's the difference? The quick answer is coconut oil contains lauric acid, known to help lower cholesterol levels. Lesson? Taco Bell—bad. Coconut oil—good.

Other Oils

I'm pretty low-key when it comes to cooking, sticking with ghee, extra-virgin olive oil, and coconut oil for almost all my baking, sauté, and dressing needs. However, there's a world of oils out there, so feel free to experiment with tastes. Other fatty friends in the Paleo world of oils include walnut, macadamia, avocado, and flax seed oils.

Avocados

If there is such a thing as the perfect food, the avocado may get my vote. There was a time back in my calorie-counting days when I would gasp in horror at the very idea of eating guacamole. "Do you have any idea how *fattening* that is?" I would ask. Thank heavens those dark days are over. Yours should be, too. And if that's the case, bring on the guac! Full of antioxidants, low in sugar, a great source of vitamins K1, B9, and C, and chock-full of energy in the form of fat, avocados are the rock star of the Paleo world. As if that's not enough, avocados help our bodies absorb nutrients, making them the perfect accompaniment to any meal.

Nuts and Seeds

Nuts and seeds are Paleo-friendly. (Pause for cheers and applause.) However, nuts are sneaky. Chances are I'm not going to accidentally plow through half a can of ghee. The same can't be said for leaving me alone with a jar of cashews. Definitely enjoy a handful of nuts each day as a snack, but do monitor your intake, especially if you're using PV to lose weight. Feel free to mix and match among the following:

Almonds	Pine nuts
Cashews	Pumpkin seeds (pepitas)
Hazelnuts	Sunflower seeds
Macadamia nuts	Walnuts
Pecans	

Note: Be wary of nuts on salads in restaurants. A salad with "tossed pecans" usually means tossed candied pecans. Same for walnuts, etc. It's easy enough to ask the server to hold the candied nuts and toss a few plain ones in there.

Eggs

Leave the egg-white omelet behind. For those of you eating eggs (and I strongly recommend you do), the yolk is where the money's at. The yolk is host to the many nutrients found in eggs, including vitamins A, B6, B12, C, D, E, and K, and is also a source of calcium, iron, folate, and zinc. It's not uncommon for me to eat as many as five to seven eggs a day. That's right. A *day*. We've been brainwashed to think of eggs, and especially the yolks, as cholesterol-producing nightmares. Not true. Eggs from pasture-raised chickens are also higher in vitamins than conventional eggs are, so if possible and within your budget, do seek them out.

Fish

I know this isn't for everyone, but if you do eat fish, go for the fatty ones—salmon, trout, and mackerel come to mind. Smaller fish like sardines, anchovies, and herring are great for snacks or to add some much-needed healthy, flavorful fat to a salad.

THE TRUTH ABOUT CHOLESTEROL

Let's talk about the elephant in the room: cholesterol. Try telling people you eat five eggs a day and watch them scramble (ha ha—get it?) to hand you their cardiologist's number. (The fact that they *have* a cardiologist should tell you something about their diet.)

Okay, moment of truth. It took me a while to embrace my love of eggs and fats. In general, I was terrified of adding fats to my diet for fear of gaining weight. With eggs, I couldn't see past the formula I'd been fed for years that egg whites were good, egg yolks were bad. After all, 1,000 anorexic-looking, egg-white-omelet-ordering movie stars can't be wrong. Or can they?

Here's the dish on cholesterol. *Dietary* cholesterol, which is what we're talking about when we talk about egg yolks, doesn't impact blood cholesterol. In fact, adding dietary cholesterol (the healthy kind) to your diet can actually help keep your blood cholesterol levels in check. Why? You're feeding your body healthy cholesterol so it doesn't feel required to make the bad stuff.

When it comes to fat and the fear of weight gain, repeat after me: Fat fills me up. Fat fills me up. Fat fills me up. In fact, one of the biggest "dieting" mistakes people make is cutting the fat from their diets. This leaves them with little to no energy for their workouts, they're almost constantly hungry, their joints ache, and they're in a mental fog as well. That's a hard row to hoe to lose some weight. The healthy fats above will give you energy, lubricated joints, and mental clarity and keep you feeling satiated after a meal. If that's not enough, the very presence of fat will help you absorb nutrients from the many fruits and vegetables you're eating. Win-win.

Fruit: The Secret Saboteur of Weight Loss?

Eat more fruits and vegetables.

Every diet in the world promotes replacing unhealthy food with healthier options like fresh fruits and vegetables. The Paleo diet and the Paleo Vegetarian diet are no exception. A handful of plump, fresh, antioxidant-boosting blueberries for a midmorning snack? Yes, please. Fruits are a quick and easy on-the-go food that taste good and can satisfy the urge for something sweet.[15] Too much of a good thing has its drawbacks, however, and fruit is no exception.

Years ago, a friend shared with me a diet that was heavily based on fast-food meats and cheese (I know, right?) but didn't allow fruit. As in, zero fruit. Zip. Nada. My incredulousness was matched only by my outrage at how yet another "miracle diet" was hoodwinking innocent people like my wanting-to-believe friend.

"There is no way that completely eliminating an entire major food group like *fruit* can be good for you," I informed her, perhaps somewhat haughtily.

"How is that any different than you wiping out an entire food group by not eating meat?" she countered.

"Well, that's…you're taking out of context…It's accepted that, I mean—hey, at least I won't get scurvy on my diet!"

Flash forward to the present, and I owe my friend an apology. While I'll never understand how a diet can get away with promoting

---

15 Once I was fully Paleo and fat-burning instead of sugar-burning, I was at a friend's house and ate a sliced strawberry offered to me. It tasted so sweet, I accused my friend of dipping it in sugar. She hadn't, but that's how much your taste buds are going to bloom. Eating foods as simple as fresh fruit feels like you've won the golden ticket into Willy Wonka's candy factory.

people to eat fast "food," it turns out there is something to weight loss and the no fruit thing.

Before you panic that I'm going to ban fruit, let me put your fears to rest. My favorite treat in life is a banana smeared in almond butter. I will not give that up. Ever. But for those interested in weight loss, too much fructose (fruit sugar) can undermine your goal. How much fruit is too much and how much is just right? Good question. Let's discuss.

THE GOAL: FAT BURNING VERSUS SUGAR BURNING

As has hopefully become clear by now, sugar is the enemy of any Paleo-based diet, as well as anyone trying to lose weight. It inflames the body and promotes weight gain. And to your body, a sugar hit is a sugar hit.

For weight loss, the guideline is you want to keep your sugars at or below 20 grams a day. That's not a lot when you consider that a banana has almost 16 grams of sugar and a medium apple has 14. Dried peaches? Forty-four grams. (I just blew your mind, I know.)

The point being, whether you eat fresh pineapple or a bag of Skittles, your insulin levels will skyrocket and that excess sugar in your blood is going to be converted to fat. To add insult to injury, many fruits are also high in carbohydrates, something that needs to be limited for weight loss.

FIBER WON'T MAKE SUGAR GO AWAY

"But what about the fiber?" I hear you asking. "I'm eating fiber when I eat fruit, so that's healthy, right?"

Please understand that I'm not saying fruit is unhealthy. And if it comes down to a choice between the pineapple and the Skittles, I will always push the pineapple. What I am saying, however, is that when you're trying to lose weight, the number-one thing you need to do isn't calorie count or exercise more or starve yourself. The number-one thing you need to do is reduce or limit your sugar intake. Period.

A diet heavy in fruit doesn't allow for this. The fiber present with fructose in fruits does slow the absorption of sugar into the bloodstream, but it doesn't completely negate it. We've still got to deal with those pesky insulin surges that, once they abate, leave us feeling droopy and lethargic and—upsettingly—hungry. And not just hungry, but sugar-craving hungry. Having had too much sugar, our bodies are giving us the SOS signal to SEND MORE SUGAR. Thus starts a vicious cycle that goes something like this: sugar leaves our bloodstream, so our body tells us it's hungry because it's craving sugar, so we eat sugar (healthy sugar, like an apple), so we're on a sugar high, so we crash, so the hunger kicks in again.

How much fruit is okay? Please don't hate me for saying this, but it really depends on the person. Men sometimes seem to tolerate fruit better than women (i.e., they can eat it and keep the weight off) but that doesn't hold true across the board. Whether you eat fruit and what kind and how much depends on your goals, your activity level, and whether or not you've made the transition from sugar-burning to fat-burning.

A common mistake for dieters turning Paleo or Paleo Vegetarian is to eat fruit as a substitute for the foods they're missing, namely grains. But while grabbing an apple at breakfast, a banana as a midmorning snack, melon at lunch, berries as another snack, and grilled pineapple at dinner *sounds* healthy, eating like that is going to send your body into a sugar tailspin that will pack on the pounds. It's also going to leave you frustrated, feeling like you're doing everything right (it's an apple, for God's sake!) but not seeing the results you desire.

AVOID FRUIT FOR THE MOMENT, NOT FOREVER

There's only one way to find out what level of fruit your body can handle and still maintain to lose weight and that's to experiment. If you're seeking to lose weight, avoid fruit for the short haul. I promise you, you'll live. I've gone years limiting myself to a piece or two of fruit *a week* and suffered no adverse health effects. And lest you think I speak for everyone, you can go on any Paleo website and chat with scads of people who, for the most part, avoid fruits as well.

If ditching fruit entirely strikes you as too extreme, limit fruit to a small amount each day, such as a handful of berries, which offer the best chance for a low insulin response. Berries are also packed with antioxidants and are nutritionally dense.

Some fruits to definitely avoid for weight loss due to their high sugar content include mangos, melons, pineapple, grapes, figs, dates, bananas (sob—my favorite!), and kiwi. Also avoid most dried fruits (did you read the thing above about the peaches?) which are high in sugar with minimal nutritional value.

Once you've gone without fruit and are following a PV diet at least 80 percent of the time and are seeing weight loss, play around with adding fruit back into your diet. Start off with lower fructose fruit like berries and work up to others like an apple or grapefruit or grapes. If the weight starts coming back on, you'll know you need to cut back.

FRUIT JUICE AND SMOOTHIES

I don't know what marketing firm was responsible for the masterful trick of making Americans think smoothies are healthy but he or she deserves to be crowned. As a general rule—no, wait. Not as a general rule. Let's just put it out there *as a rule*: avoid smoothies.

They're filled with fruit which, as we've already seen, is a barrier to weight loss. But almost every smoothie has added ingredients like honey or peanut butter or syrups or just added sugar to sweeten them even more.

Perusing the online nutritional counter for one national smoothie chain, I see that a "Low-Carb Banana" smoothie has 39 grams of sugar. And a "Slim and Trim Chocolate" smoothie has 48 grams. For weight loss, we're aiming for 20 grams per day. Two sips of one of these "healthy" smoothies and you've reached your sugar max for the day. Avoid them.

Also, unless you know for a fact that you can tolerate loads of fruit and not gain weight, throw away your juicer. You don't need that much fruit in one serving. And never, ever, ever buy fruit juice, also known as the devil's elixir. (Okay, I made that up.) Expect anywhere from 20 to 40 grams of sugar in an eight-ounce glass. Not worth it.

FRUIT IS NOT THE ENEMY

For all that I've said to vilify fruit, it really is our friend. Fruits can help satisfy a sweet tooth. A handful of blueberries at night after dinner takes the place of a big, sticky, overly sweet dessert that would leave you feeling bloated and gross. Instead you get your taste of something sweet and walk away from the table feeling good about yourself and your choices. (My advice on this is to make sure, before indulging, that you know you have the ability to walk away.)

As we'll see in the athlete's section (page 187), fruit also has a place and purpose in our diet around workouts. And a final tip, some people find that eating fruit with a protein helps keep the weight off, versus eating a piece of fruit on its own.

Again, nothing here is to say that fruit makes you fat. But what it can do is impede the goal of turning you into a fat-burning machine instead of a sugar-burning machine. That's why it's suggested (not mandated, but suggested) that if you're in this for weight loss, you exclude or limit fruit, slowly adding it back to your diet in a controlled fashion after you've met your goal.

Chapter 7

PV Foraging at the Grocery Store: Shopping Lists, Meal Plans, and Dining Out

Grocery Shopping

To eat PV, we must cook PV. And to cook PV, we must first shop PV. Again, unless you are a junk-food vegetarian (you're not a junk-food vegetarian, are you? Please tell me you're not), your Paleo Vegetarian shopping list isn't going to look dramatically different from your prior list—minus a few grains, of course. Curious about what to buy and what to leave behind? Below are some tips to guide you through the grocery aisles and ensure you fill your cart with healthy, hearty PV staples.

PRODUCE

Here's where you'll spend the bulk of your time and your money. You know the drill here—choose a rainbow of colors and go heavy on the greens: rainbow chard, collards, kale, spinach. Grab handfuls of onions, peppers, and tomatoes, as these will be the base of a lot of your recipes. And cauliflower. Oh Lord, will you go through some cauliflower. Able to be transformed into rice or potatoes, it's like this cheap, magical food staring you in the face.

Ask questions and don't be afraid to try new things. It took me three years before I learned how to cook an eggplant dish that didn't cause an involuntary gag reflex in my spouse. (See page 164 for the recipe.) But eggplants just look so big and beautiful and purple that I kept putting them in my cart each week, much to the dismay of my husband.

Figure out what you like and then eat it like it's going out of style. I personally am a brussels sprouts whore. Can't get enough of them. I have been known to literally wipe out a store's brussels sprouts allotment in one trip. I throw them in salads, eat them for breakfast, and snack on them. If your thing is beets or asparagus or radishes, don't hold back. It's a *vegetable*. Now is not the time for restraint.

SHOP THE PERIMETER

It seems like a different lifetime when "going to the store" meant slowly pushing my cart up and down every single aisle, pausing every few feet to toss another box of pasta or bag of cereal[16] into my cart. People, I can't even *remember* the last time I went down the cookie aisle, and they could have relocated the bread and cracker aisle to Cambodia for all I know. Eating PV means eating real food, whole food, *recognizable* food, and very little of that is found in the center aisles of a grocery store. Spend your time in the outer perimeters and shop yourself into a happier, healthier life.

---

16 Why yes, generic fruit loops were a large part of my vegetarian diet, thank you very much for asking.

Remember, if you're looking to lose weight, go light on the fruit. It may look healthy to load your cart up with apples, bananas, kiwi, pineapple, mangos, and melon but that's a whole truckload of sugar just waiting to be converted into fat. If you're shedding pounds, stick with berries, as they have lower sugars and are also filled with antioxidants.

WHAT'S IN THE ATHLETE'S PV PANTRY?

Vegetables like squash, yam, beets, and sweet potatoes are all Paleo-approved and damn tasty to boot. Even if you're not an athlete, you can still feel free to enjoy these foods, but as in everything, moderation is the key. A sweet potato a day? Not if you want to lose weight. A serving of spaghetti squash with a vegetable marinara after a challenging workout? Yup.

DAIRY

Depending on if you want to go hardcore Paleo or the gentler Primal will determine how much time you spend in the dairy section. Let's talk about the two things you (may) be buying there: eggs and cheese.

Eggs

Sadly, my friends who had the chickens moved away, so I was once again left to turn to commercial establishments for eggs. I take the time to seek out pasture-raised[17] eggs. As my folksy egg carton says, "*That means raised on grass, y'all.*" I like pasture-raised

---

17 Don't confuse pasture-raised with "pasteurized." Pasteurized means heat has been used to eliminate things like the salmonella bacteria so that the eggs can be eaten raw. A lot of liquid eggs are pasteurized, whole eggs less so, but they can still be found. Note that this has to do with heating the eggs to make them safe and nothing to do with nutritional content or how the hens are raised.

for several reasons. One, it means the chickens who laid the eggs are allowed to roam free, eating happy-chicken things like bugs and grass and plants. The second reason is that pasture-raised eggs have been shown to be more nutritious, with significantly higher levels of vitamins A and E, and omega-3s. Do I cringe a bit inside every time I pay close to $9 for a carton of eggs? Yes. Do I cringe more every time I eat a conventional egg at a restaurant or a friend's home or at my mom's? (C'mon Mom—get with the program!) You bet.

Think about the circle of life when buying eggs. Conventional chickens—aside from never seeing the light of day—are fed a grain-based diet sometimes supplemented with animal byproducts and food from GMO crops. Many are injected with hormones. All that nasty stuff that goes into the chickens is going to come out at least a little bit in their eggs.

What about all the organic and omega-3-enriched eggs? Organic eggs at least have the no antibiotics or hormones thing going for them, although organic and even "cage-free" doesn't mean these chickens are living a happy life. ("Pasture-raised" is no guarantee either, but there's a much better chance of it.)

Entire books and websites are devoted to the different kinds of eggs, how the chickens who produce them are raised and cared (or not cared) for, and the different nutritional value of each. I understand $9 eggs may not be in everyone's budget, especially if you're feeding a family. But if you're able to afford them, I do believe that since you're expending all this energy to eat and live healthy, you should strive to put the healthiest foods into your body, as your budget allows. And to quote Forrest Gump, "That's all I have to say about that."

Cheese

Ah, cheese. Hard chunks, ooey-gooey stringy, served over crackers, or melted on top of a casserole…it's hard not to love such a versatile, tasty food.

Hardcore Paleo says no cheese. (I think of the soup Nazi from *Seinfeld*, only instead of "No soup for you!" it's "No cheese for you!") But Primal allows for the occasional treat of cheese. Grass-fed cheese is ideal but trust me on this—waiters are going to roll their eyes at you in most restaurants or give you a blank, non-comprehending stare if you ask them if the feta in your salad is "grass-fed." Let's just assume all cheese you would eat at a restaurant is not.

Let's also take a moment to discuss what is meant by "occasional" and "a treat." You may do well to decide up front what your own rules will be around handling cheese, if you choose to eat it. My "rules" are that I'm okay with goat cheese and feta crumbled in salads, although I do ask for it on the side and usually end up sprinkling on only about half of what they bring me. If there's a cheese tray at a party, I enjoy a thin slice or two of Gouda or any good, aged cheese. I do not keep cheese in the house and I only order it on my salads if I really, really want it. If I'm feeling "eh" about it, I skip it and save it for a day when I'm having a real craving.

Unless I'm on a cheat day (more about that later), a big slice of pizza dripping in melted mozzarella or a pot of fondue cheese is *not* considered "a treat." That's called gorging, people. Don't do it. And especially don't eat that cheap, crappy fast-food pizza cheese. If you want pizza, make a white bean crust (see page 153) and buy some organic, non-homogenized dairy at a specialty store and really indulge in the taste of a good and flavorful cheese.

As a Paleo Vegetarian, you might indulge in cheese a bit more than meat-eating Primal dieters, as most cheese does pack a wallop of protein. Just remember to keep portions small.

Other Dairy

Coffee lovers take heart. Going PV does not mean you are resigned to a lifetime of unsweetened black drudge. While Paleo bans all dairy, a Primal diet allows for some hacks, including a tiny bit of heavy cream in your coffee. Make sure it's heavy cream, as it's free of most lactose and casein. Is it super high in fat? You bet, but it's good fat that fills you up. Just don't go overboard.

I went to Starbucks a while back and ordered a coffee with just a tiny bit of heavy cream. I believe the words I used were "a smidge." I happened to watch them make my coffee and the barista must have poured almost a quarter cup of cream into my small coffee. Now when I go to Starbucks or wherever, I ask for a tablespoon of heavy cream in my coffee and then I make eye-contact with the barista and stress, "And I mean, literally, a *tablespoon* of heavy cream. No more." You have to be proactive.

What other dairy is tolerated? A staple in my life is grass-fed butter (usually available at Whole Foods) or ghee which I use to sauté vegetables and spread on toasted Paleo Bread (recipe page 155).

FROZEN FOODS

Along the far perimeter of the store you'll find the time-crunched PV eater's best friend: the frozen food aisle. Do yourself a favor: Grab a second cart and load up. Most veggies are frozen at their peak so the nutrients are locked in, plus it's often cheaper to buy frozen rather than fresh produce. And the convenience factor can't be beat. I keep bags—*bags*—of frozen veggies in the freezer in my office break room at work. I'm a stress eater, which means

I pretty much have the urge to eat all day, every day. Instead of hitting the vending machine and flinging myself into a sugar coma, I toss a bag of mixed veggies in the microwave, add a dash of red pepper flakes and munch on that.

What frozen vegetables should you buy? Any and all *so long as they are vegetables only.* Avoid any vegetables that come covered in cheese, sweet-and-sour sauce, or butter (it won't be the good, pure butter we're after). Watch out for mixed blends that contain corn (a grain), potatoes, black-eyed peas, and chickpeas.

CANNED GOODS

It's time to venture down an aisle. Canned goods aren't always as healthy as fresh or frozen options (there are more preservatives and it seems like they're sneakier about adding in extra sugar and salt) but they're still a good option for a number of foods. Here's a list of canned items to stock up on, keeping in mind to buy low-sodium and organic when possible:

- Tomato paste

- Tomato sauce

- Any type of Paleo-approved vegetable (no corn, peas, or potatoes) that floats your boat

- Water chestnuts

- Olives[18]

- Artichoke hearts (plain, not marinated)

- Low-sodium beans (black, white, pinto, kidney, chickpeas sparingly), if you're using in moderation

---

18 A fruit, but a healthy one low in sugar. Olives are high in sodium, so eat in moderation and double check the label to make sure they're free of additives. Greek olives are usually a safe bet, but explore black and green options. Avoid pimento-stuffed, but a few blue-cheese stuffed olives occasionally are delicious.

- Sun-dried tomatoes (either dry or in olive oil only; sprinkle in with scrambled eggs and in salads)

- Coconut milk—read the label and look for low sugar and no additives

- Applesauce, no sugar added, and watch for additives

- Canned pumpkin. Pumpkin is a cooking staple in many Paleo kitchens. It can be high in sugar so don't go eating it straight from the can (I've *never* done that) but Google "Paleo pumpkin recipes" and you'll find everything from muffins and pancakes (grain-free, of course) to soups and chili. Pumpkin is a great natural sweetener in recipes, and for people who work out a lot and need more energy, pumpkin, along with other squashes or yams/sweet potatoes, is a great source of carbs.

For the pescatarian Paleo Vegetarians:

- Water-packed tuna

- Wild-caught salmon

- Sardines

What about soups? Sorry—most canned soups are decidedly non-PV-friendly, containing sugar, dairy, corn, rice, soy, and a long list of unpronounceable additives and preservatives. Soup is a great Paleo option if you make it yourself, which is why we've included a few yummy options in the recipe section. When you make soup, triple the recipe and freeze it in quart-size bags. Then, on days you're stressed for time, it's a matter of just pulling a bag out of the freezer and letting it thaw until lunchtime at work for a healthy, delicious, PV-approved meal.

OILS AND DRESSINGS

Embrace the reality that there is no ready-made dressing on the shelf that's PV-friendly. The sugar content of most salad dressings is high enough that your average honey mustard ought to be considered a viable treat to give out on Halloween, right next to the Snickers and peanut butter cups. (Good luck explaining that to a five-year-old, however.) Either make your own dressings, or if you're lazy like me, carry around extra-virgin olive oil packets and just use that, sometimes with a little balsamic vinegar as well.

Given all the cooking you'll be doing, it's wise to stock up on Paleo-approved oils and fats. These include:

- Coconut oil—Great at high temperatures, and life opened up for me once I had my first taste of fresh-from-the farm green beans roasted and drizzled in coconut oil. YUM.

- Olive oil and extra-virgin olive oil

- Macadamia oil—A fun alternative to coconut oil.

- Avocado oil—If you don't like the taste of avocados, don't do this diet. (Kidding. But no, seriously…)

- Grass-fed butter or ghee

DRY AND BAKING GOODS

Now that you have so much open pantry space having cleared out all those bags of rice, barley, spelt, and oats (you did toss them, right?), you've got plenty of room for the good stuff, such as:

- Almond meal

- Coconut flour

- Coconut aminos[19]

---

19 Coconut aminos is a Paleo-friendly alternative to soy sauce. It's made from coconut sap with a little sea salt added in. Great for Asian dishes and stir-fries.

- Vegetable stock (read the ingredient list again to avoid sugars and additives, or make your own)
- Nuts (almonds, macadamias, cashews, hazelnuts... no peanuts!)
- Coffee and tea
- Beans (if you're using in moderation)
- Maple syrup—the real stuff. Just say no to Aunt Jemima.
- Applesauce with no sugar or additives
- Herbs and spices

BECOME A LABEL READER

Actually, become a label *scrutinizer*. There are so many foods out there that at first glance appear to be Paleo-friendly but upon a closer read, turn out to have vegetable oil or soy or sugars. Just because a product touts itself as "All Natural!" on the label doesn't mean it's true. Even things like "artificial colors and flavorings" are reason to pause before purchasing. Do you know what ingredients go into "artificial flavors"? I don't. But I'm guessing they're not Paleo.

What follows is a short, non-comprehensive list of some of the more common ingredients that indicate the presence of wheat, soy, sugar, or corn. As always, a good rule of thumb is that if you don't recognize it and can't pronounce it, don't eat it.

- Barley malt syrup
- Bleached flour
- Cane crystals
- Corn sweetener
- Corn syrup

- Dehydrated cane juice

- Dextrin

- Dexatrose

- Evaporated cane juice

- Fruit juice concentrate

- Hydrolyzed vegetable protein (HVP)

- Malt or malt syrup

- Maltodextrin

- Miso

- Modified food or gum starch

- Monosaccharide

- MSG

- Polysaccharide

- Rice syrup

- Sorbitol

- Tamari

- Tempeh

- Textured soy flour (TSF)/textured soy protein (TSP)/ textured vegetable protein (TVP)

- Tofu

- Wheat protein

- Xantham gum

Also, don't get thrown by items labeled "gluten-free." Remember, you're entering a *grain-free* world. The majority of the gluten-free items on the market are still rice or oats based and most of them contain an appalling amount of sugar, sodium, and a list of ingredients that requires a masters in chemistry to decipher.

PREPACKAGED "PALEO" FOOD

Now that Paleo has gone mainstream, there are industries being built around providing would-be Paleoists (or Paleo Vegetarians) with either quick-and-easy Paleo foods on the go or food replacements for the items people tend to miss most, like snack bars, cereals, breads, pancakes, brownies, etc.

Most true Paleoists come down on the side that the whole point of eating Paleo is to eat clean, whole foods and that if you're having to rely on these prepackaged items, you're not truly Paleo and it's unlikely you've fully converted to a fat-burning rather than sugar-burning machine.

I agree with this camp. Based on my experience, I *gained* weight when I added prepackaged Paleo foods to my diet. However, I went overboard. I was so excited to find bread and cereal and brownies that I thought were "safe" that I ended up eating those foods to the exclusion of most everything else. I've learned to cut back and now I don't see anything wrong with having an occasional Paleo bar or cookie, so long as the majority of my diet remains strong in vegetables and other whole foods.

I will say that I am a loyal consumer of the Paleo bread found at JulianBakery.com. Sometimes you just want a sandwich. Or toast. This is just my experience, but I find that when I eat the bread on a daily basis, I start to gain weight. If I limit myself to a couple of slices a week, I'm happy and I don't notice any negative effects.

I'd suggest you hold off on ordering or experimenting with any of these prepackaged foods for the first 30 days after you transition to PV. Get a handle on eating PV the way it's meant to be eaten—lots of veggies and some beans, and colorful whole-food flavor combinations. Then if you find you're really missing a certain something and having a Paleo option for it available would help keep you on track, go ahead and try it. Do monitor your weight and how you feel when eating the item and pull back if you notice either a) you have a sudden sugar craving after eating the food, indicating it may have hidden sugars, or b) your weight starts to creep back up.

WHAT ABOUT ORGANIC?

Should you be buying organic foods? Lord, I don't know. Kidding. Well, only kind of kidding. There's so much vitriolic discussion these days about the benefits/pseudobenefits of organic that it can be hard to know where to come down on the issue.

What remains steadfast is that it's always good to buy the "Dirty Dozen" foods organic. The Environmental Working Group (EWG) at Ewg.org/foodnews puts the Dirty Dozen together, and while most items on the list remain consistent, there are occasional substitutions. The most recent 2014 list of the most pesticide-laden produce on the market includes:

- apples
- celery
- cherry tomatoes
- cucumbers
- grapes
- nectarines (imported)
- peaches
- potatoes
- snap peas (imported)
- spinach
- strawberries
- sweet bell peppers

The EWG also releases the "Clean 15" list, those foods with the lowest pesticide ratings. These include:

- asparagus
- avocados
- cabbage
- cantaloupe
- cauliflower
- eggplant
- grapefruit
- kiwi
- mangos
- onions
- papayas
- pineapples

- sweet corn
- sweet peas (frozen)
- sweet potatoes

Given my druthers, everything I eat would be organic. However, that's rarely practical from both an availability and monetary standpoint. Do I think one salad of nonorganic spinach is going to harm me? Nah. But given that I eat a—what's the scientific term for it? Oh yes—a *butt load* of spinach each week in salads and stir fries, yes, I try to buy organic. I do think quantity counts.

If you can't buy organic, a really good rinse of your vegetables will help at least cut down on the pesticides present. And I still think a pesticide-laden cherry tomato is still better for me than a bag of Doritos, any day.

I'm a big fan of buying food from my local farmer's market as well. It's almost always healthier, fresher, and cheaper than the stuff at the grocery store, and personally, I like supporting local farmers.

Dining Out

Does eating PV mean you never get to dine out again? Not at all. With a little planning (and willingness to be *that* person at the table who special orders), you can eat everywhere from fast food to Mexican restaurants, Indian to Chinese eateries.

That being said, please understand that even though you can find options at many of these restaurants, they're typically less than ideal. You may have to sacrifice perfection and eat vegetables that are cooked in non-PV-approved oils, or eat beans as your primary protein source, or even (gasp!) break code and eat a baked potato. So long as you're not eating out constantly and making these choices a consistent part of your life, one or two servings a month of close-but-not-quite PV food from restaurants is not going to ruin you.

Obviously (and especially if you're following a PV diet in order to lose weight) the healthiest option is always to prepare your own food at home. That way there's no question what oils were used, that no hidden sugars were added, and that the food wasn't loaded with enough sodium to choke a camel. (Just saying.)

Still, if you have kids or a job or, I don't know, *a life,* it's almost inevitable that you're going to be dragged out to McDonald's or find yourself seated at a birthday luncheon at a Mexican restaurant while your coworker wears the birthday sombrero and is serenaded by staff who *keep bringing chips and salsa* to the table. In times like these, it will serve you well to know ahead of time what you will and will not eat.

If possible, try to limit your eating out the first month or two you're following the PV diet. The way of eating will still be new to you, and it's easy to get frustrated or tempted by all the delicious-looking "but-I-can't-have-it" foods in restaurants that you used to enjoy. Change is coming though. America is awakening to the fact that sugar is making us fat and—quite literally—killing us. The hidden menu at Panera Bread is surprisingly Paleo-friendly (although, unfortunately, given all the steak, chicken, and turkey options, not PV-friendly) and a number of other restaurants are slowly following suit with hidden or "alternative" menus. Why healthy, delicious choices must be hidden from the public view is beyond me, but that's a discussion for another time.

So let's dig in. What can you eat and where, and is there any chance at all it will come in a Happy Meal box? (Answer: negative.) Obviously we can't cover every restaurant, but what's here can serve as a guide for those times you find yourself staring at a menu and debating whether sweet potato fries can be considered Paleo.[20]

---

20 Sorry, no. Most sweet potato fries are prepared in vegetable oil and dusted with cinnamon-sugar.

The smartest thing you can do to ensure you stick to the PV diet when dining out is to look at the menu ahead of time online and decide, from the safety of your home or desk, what you'll be eating. Willpower weakens at the moment of decision but having a predetermined path seems to keep many people *on* the path. Good luck, and happy ordering!

MEXICAN RESTAURANTS

Thanks to America's love affair with fajitas, Mexican restaurants have an abundance of fresh veggies on hand, not to mention they're rolling in black beans. Ask for a fajita salad (not served in the fried tortilla bowl unless you have more willpower than me), have them bring you black beans on the side to sprinkle on top of the salad, and ask what type of oil the veggies are cooked in and if there's any chance they could specially prepare some for you in either butter or olive oil. Also be sure to load up your salad with avocado and even some of the salsa, especially if it's fresh, with big chunks of tomatoes in it.

CHINESE RESTAURANTS

You can eat PV at most Chinese restaurants, but you'll most likely need to bid the buffet—and all the fried goodness on it—good-bye. Instead, ask for steamed vegetables. It's okay to indulge in a little white rice if this is going to be a main meal (or, even better, if you're eating right after a workout). Just make sure you ask that anything they prepare for you be made with no MSG. As for soups, egg drop and hot and sour soups are okay options as long as they're not made with cornstarch—and good luck getting a server who has any idea if they're made with that or not.

INDIAN RESTAURANTS

Indian food is traditionally predominantly vegetarian and therefore offers a wider array of vegetarian options than most other cuisines. But what, you may ask (or at least, I ask) is the point of eating Indian food without naan bread to sop up the remnants of your meal? Well, the point is that even without the bread, Indian food is very tasty, very healthy, and typically cooked to order. Indian chefs also do *amazing* things with cauliflower and spices that will leave you drooling and completely happy with your meal.

ITALIAN RESTAURANTS

Eating out Italian can sometimes feel more challenging just because it was likely your go-to place before with friends who wanted to make sure their vegetarian friend had something to eat. Since you're no longer filling your plate with pasta, what next? Depending on the restaurant, eating PV at an Italian eatery is either difficult to impossible (Pizza Hut) or pretty easy (mom-and-pop authentic Italian spots). There are also in-between places like Olive Garden that, while far from ideal, can get you a meal. My favorite trick at Italian restaurants is to get the pasta toppings I always have (marinara sauce with grilled veggies, for example) and ask for it over grilled eggplant or zucchini. Asking for toppings over wilted spinach is another option. I've been to a few places that have a steak-and-veggie kabob that I've asked them to make for me, hold the steak, extra veggies.

STEAK HOUSES

Surprisingly, I've found steak houses to be the most accommodating to the PV diet. You can order a plate of vegetables that includes a baked sweet potato, steamed broccoli and cauliflower, sautéed spinach with roasted garlic, and vegetables of the day. They usually have exceptional salads with all the good stuff—radishes and carrots and cucumber and noncandied nuts like pecans or walnuts. If you eat dairy, ask for a little goat cheese on your salad. Steak houses also use real butter, so ask for some in a side dish and dunk your veggies in it or pat some on your sweet potato, pop open a bottle of red wine with friends, and enjoy.

BREAKFAST PLACES

Breakfast places like IHOP and Denny's are some of my favorite restaurants to eat at. Nothing says Paleo Vegetarian like an omelet the size of your face. I ask what the eggs and vegetables are cooked in—requesting if need be that they replace the canola or vegetable oil with butter—and then go to town. My omelet orders are legendary among friends. *Reminder: Do not order the egg-white omelet. Yolk is healthy fat and it's filling, so go whole-egg.* Then pile in all the fresh veggies you love—broccoli, peppers, mushrooms, spinach, artichoke hearts, sun-dried tomatoes, black olives, jalapeno, avocado…the list goes on. If you're eating beans, do a Mexican omelet with black beans and salsa. A small side of blueberries or strawberries (it won't be on the menu, but ask for them—they use them to make pancakes and can stick them in a dish for you) is a sweet tooth–satisfying dessert.

FAST FOOD

For better or worse (and no question it's for worse), fast food is a part of most of our lives. Our coworkers eat there, our kids beg us to eat there, and even our spouses put in the occasional plea. While eating at the places below should not become a habit, there are workarounds.

Chipotle

Friend of both Paleoists and vegetarians, Chipotle offers one of the easiest and tastiest ways to eat out and stick to the PV diet. Go for the salad bowl and load it up with veggies and guacamole. Add in black beans for protein, but avoid the pinto beans as they're cooked with bacon. Technically, the fajita vegetables aren't Paleo as they're sautéed in soybean oil, but unless you're eating Chipotle every day for most meals, one serving of these vegetables for a lunch out won't do you in. Skip the vinaigrette as it's made with honey and rice bran oil, and instead use one of the fresh salsas as a dressing.

Panera Bread

Often touted as "healthy" fast food, it's actually pretty hard to find PV food at Panera. That's due to a high amount of sugars and oils in most of their foods, including the "healthy" soup options. Panera's hidden menu does offer some great options for Paleoists that can be modified for PV. They have a number of healthy salads that can be made PV-friendly by asking to hold the meat (and egg, if need be). In that case, you're paying close to $9 for pretty much lettuce, onion, cucumber, and half an avocado, but at least you'll have something to eat. If you do eat eggs, ask them to skip the meat but give you an extra hard-boiled egg. For breakfast, I've asked them to give me just the egg (or "egg-like") patty they use on breakfast sandwiches as a side.[21] The other good thing about Panera's hidden menu is that it comes with a small, self-contained packet of extra-virgin olive oil. Sometimes I'll order the Greek salad (which does have feta cheese—Primal, not Paleo) and have them

---

21 Note: It will take two Panera workers and a manager seven minutes to figure out how to ring this up.

hold the non-PV Greek dressing[22] and give me the little packet of the EVOO instead.

Cracker Barrel

I'm not sure what their vegetables are cooked in, but at least you can get a plate of nothing but vegetables at Cracker Barrel. If you eat fish, the spicy baked (not fried) catfish is an option, and if you eat eggs you can get a big ol' plateful of fried or scrambled eggs with a side of collard greens or fruit. Cracker Barrel also offers steamed broccoli and a baked sweet potato that can make for a filling meal when combined with a side salad. Pull up a chair, y'all.

Taco Bell

Eat anything you want. Ha ha! Yeah, there's nothing here for us, people. Move along.

McDonald's/Wendy's/Burger King

I love a challenge. Okay, really the only remotely PV items you're going to find at these places are the salads. The chicken salads, if you're willing to pay more and pick the chicken off, typically have more good stuff on them like cucumber and carrots and tomatoes. Just make sure to avoid the croutons and, again, you're way ahead of the game if you bring your own dressing. Unfortunately, eating these salads with no protein isn't going to be filling but if you HAVE to eat at one of these venues, at least you can appear not to be antisocial by eating a little something with the group. McDonald's offers apple slices as a kid's side that you can order. Also, a baked potato from Wendy's with broccoli (no cheese) is

---

22 Now's a good time to mention that you should get in the habit of carrying olive oil and vinegar with you when eating out at fast-food restaurants. You can get a salad almost anywhere but none—repeat, *none*—of the dressings, including the vinaigrettes, are PV.

another decent option. White potatoes are one of those foods that waver on the Paleo line. They're a dense carbohydrate source and they do spike blood sugar, but they're more nutritionally empty than they are nutritionally harmful. When baked not fried, they're an acceptable option if there's nothing else to eat.

GENERAL TIPS FOR EATING OUT

That's pretty much it for the restaurants. Now let's look at a few notes on eating out in general that will make your life easier.

PAY THE EXTRA CASH. Those huge omelets I get? The first three ingredients are free and after that it's 50 cents a veggie. Restaurants may also charge you extra for special orders (not usually, but some do). You may have to order three grilled chicken salads at a fast-food place to pick off chicken and have enough lettuce left to make one decent meal. It's not fun, but I pay it. Wouldn't you rather be out an extra $6 and have a meal you enjoy?

BE ASSERTIVE. This brings us to the not-so-fun part of dining out. You get to be "that guy" or "that girl" that takes an hour to order as you drill the waiter on what's in the food, how it's cooked, where it's sourced, and if there's any chance it may have come in contact with a peanut (kidding). It takes some chutzpah. But stick to your guns. That doesn't mean being rude. I typically joke with the waitstaff before I place my order that I get to be their challenging diner of the night and wish them luck. It lets them know that I'm aware I'm a pain in their arse, but I also don't let them off the hook.

DON'T APOLOGIZE FOR YOUR PV DIET. Waitstaff see it all: nut allergies, food sensitivities, Weight Watchers, vegans, fruititarians, calorie counters, people who only eat white food, etc. They don't have the time during a busy shift to stand there and listen to the details of what you can and can't eat on your diet in an all-encompassing overview. Simply look at the menu, figure out your best options, ask some questions, and provide general guidelines as necessary, such as, "I'd prefer not to eat anything cooked in vegetable oil—is it an option to prepare some vegetables in butter?"

ASK ABOUT OFF-MENU ITEMS. The waitstaff know the menu inside and out. Ask for their help. "I'm trying to piece together a meal of just vegetables but I'm tired of salads—what do you suggest?"

SUBSTITUTE. Substitutions are the name of the game. Look over the menu and notice what ingredients are used in what dishes. For example, maybe there's a fish served over a bed of rice with sautéed spinach. Boom—now you know they have sautéed spinach. Look over the steak, fish, and pasta options just to see what ingredients are being used. You know the restaurant has them in-house and you can ask for them as sides. I've created my own meals, like asking for the veggie marinara from a pasta dish to be served over the baked cauliflower from a steak dish and served with a side of artichoke hearts and olives I saw as a topping on a fish dish. Yum.

TIP WELL. Make no mistake. You are a hassle. You will be polite and considerate, but chances are you'll still have your server running in and out of the kitchen at least twice to check on how certain foods are prepared. When your waiter delivers the food, your friends will hear "Enjoy," while you will hear, "Did I get that right?" Behind the scenes, the chefs are griping to the waiter about having to specially prepare your handful of veggies. Be considerate and tip well—very well. Especially if the waitstaff went above and beyond (which I'm surprised how often they do) to accommodate your "weird" dietary needs.

I'm also a fan of calling the manager over at the end of a good meal to call out the wonderfulness of my server and the chef. Kind words go a long way and will make your waiter or waitress's night, their manager's night, and hopefully the chef's night. They may also remember you when you return and be more inclined to be helpful once again.

RESEARCH AHEAD OF TIME. The best defense is a good offense. If you're going out with friends or family, check out the online menu of the place you're heading prior to being seated. If you're not sure there's something for you there, call ahead of time. Even for Wendy's, Burger King, or McDonald's, look the menu over ahead of time and have a plan about what you can order or—even better—if you know you're going there, bring a few extras of your own, like a bag of sliced veggies you can pour over a salad to make a meal.

AVOID BUFFETS. Most buffets are fried-food and sugar havens. Indian, Chinese, pizza, or breakfast bar, your best bet for getting a PV meal will always be to order off the menu.

SAVE THE "I'M ALLERGIC" PLOY FOR ONLY THE DIREST CIRCUMSTANCES. I'm not proud of this, but most Paleoists I know have, at one time or another, pulled the "I have allergies" claim on why their food had to be prepared a certain way. Do waiters and chefs believe people are actually allergic to canola oil? I have no idea. But they do take gluten allergies seriously and will work with you to avoid any form of gluten in your meal.

Note: Use discretion with this tactic. You shouldn't have to lie about your dietary choices, and you also may have the experience I did where I was in an upscale Italian restaurant with friends, lied and said I had a gluten allergy, and watched the well-trained staff go into a three-alarm alert. All my food was prepared in a separate kitchen they had set up just for gluten-free cooking, the waiter told me about her sister who had similar issues and wanted to compare notes with me on how I discovered my allergy. Needless to say, I felt guilty and foolish for the ruse. The only reason to pull it out is, well, probably never. Maybe if the waitstaff is resisting you, but it's probably better to just eat a little non-Paleo food that night and make a note not to return to that restaurant again.

SALADS ARE YOUR FRIEND. You may have noticed that a lot of what you'll be eating out is salads. It sounds boring, and in cases like fast-food joints, it is. (I don't know about you, but I'm at a point in my life where I find iceberg lettuce insulting.) But—and as vegetarians you probably already know this—salads can be some of the most inventive cuisines out there. Think BAS: Big Ass Salad. Throw vegetables on in different combinations and the tastes change. Make it a challenge to take a nonhealthy restaurant and see what flavor combinations you can come up with there. It doesn't happen often (because I'm surrounded by meat-loving friends), but there have been times when everyone at the table oohs and ahhs as my meal is set before me, my healthy sea of greens and vegetables a delicious contrast to the piles of greasy food congealing on their plates.

EAT NON-PV. What is this? Blasphemy? No, it's reality. Eating out is not going to be an everyday occurrence, so why not enjoy the occasional times you do go out? I don't mean you entirely go crazy, but if you eat a meal that's 80 percent PV perfect, that's close enough. Maybe your cheat is some steamed white rice to go under your veggies, or a baked Idaho potato because a sweet potato wasn't available. Or you went for the Indian buffet even though most of the vegetables are cooked in soybean or sunflower oil, and you ate the rice. Again, as long as this is an occasional occurrence (maybe once a month or once every couple of weeks), it's not life shattering. Food is a social aspect of your life. Don't get so uptight over what you can and can't have that you forget to enjoy the experience of eating and spending time with the people you're with.

SEEK OUT LOCAL. As time goes by, you'll come to know which restaurants in your area are more PV-friendly than others. Your best bet is almost always nonchain restaurants where managers and staff work a little harder to accommodate guests. Does this mean you can never eat at Olive Garden or Red Lobster again? Nope. But local restaurants in general are usually more accommodating as they're seeking to establish relationships and attract loyal customers—which you'll soon become if they deliver a fantastic PV meal.

Chapter 8

Cheat Days and the 80/20 Principle

Is it possible to have your Paleo-forbidden bread and eat it too? This chapter may just hold the key for many people to making Paleo Vegetarianism a sustainable diet for life.

Question: What is it we don't like about diets?

Answer: Restriction.

The minute we commit to a diet, it seems like the food around us becomes one great, big tempting world of "NO." Having to continually walk through this world and operate in a state of denial takes a toll on our mental and emotional stores—which in turn can take a toll on our bodies. Frankly, it's depressing not to be able to eat what we want, especially when so many people around us are doing just that. No one wants to operate in that space forever, but so many of us don't see any other option.

What if I told you there was another way. What if instead of a world of "Nope, not now, not ever," you lived in a world of "Not now, but yes later."

Welcome to the concept of cheat days and 80/20 eating.

Cheat Days

The first time I heard of a cheat day was while reading *The 4-Hour Body* by Tim Ferriss, author of the worldwide bestseller *The 4-Hour Workweek*. Ferriss is an admitted body hacker, constantly testing and trying out new ways to push, pump up, and improve the body with the most minimal amount of effort involved. The Slow-Carb Diet recommended in his book was actually my intro into the world of Paleo eating. The two plans are similar in that there is a strong emphasis in both on eating vegetables and nontoxin, grass-fed beef and pasture-raised meat as the base. The main differences are that, unlike Paleo, the Slow-Carb Diet forbids all fruit but encourages the consumption of beans for a "slow-carb" energy source, making the diet much more vegetarian-friendly. Ferris also encourages the weekly allowance of—drum roll please—*the cheat day!*

Ferriss advocates one day a week where you throw caution to the wind and eat whatever the hell you want. Pizza, beer, Snickers… unwrap it, bring it on, eat it up. No calorie counting, no restrictions. Any food in any quantity is fair game.

Why do cheat days work? Aren't you just undoing a week's worth of hard work and sacrifice when you sit down to a jelly doughnut and a keg of chocolate milk on Sunday? I'm not a scientist or nutritionist, nor am I body hacker like Ferriss. All I can offer is that I've seen the cheat day work for me, and that Ferriss and his legions of followers swear by it. Per Ferriss, this is why the cheat day works for you instead of against you:

> Paradoxically, dramatically spiking caloric intake in this way once per week increases fat loss by ensuring that your metabolic rate (thyroid function, etc.) doesn't downregulate

from extended caloric restriction.[23] That's right: eating pure crap can help you lose fat. Welcome to Utopia.

I find cheat days to be the most effective means around for controlling my food intake during the week. I have a wicked sweet tooth and will get a craving for, let's say, a Reese's Peanut Butter Cup. Instead of telling myself, "No, you can't have that," I tell myself, "You can have as many of them as you want on Saturday." Oddly, that does the trick. Or maybe it's not so odd. Realistically, if you tell yourself you can never have pizza (or whatever your favorite non-PV food is) again, do you believe what you're saying? Or do you know that there's a really good chance that at some point, probably sooner rather than later, you're going to have a craving and the idea of "I can never eat this again" is not going to sit well with you? And so what happens? You rebel, go off on a binge, and spend the next 24 hours feeling terrible about yourself and your inability to just say no. Wouldn't it be more productive—and make you feel better about yourself—to exert control during the week and have a plan for how to "cheat"?

Cheat days are essentially controlled binges. Do you *have* to participate in cheat days? Absolutely not. In fact, some people prefer to reduce the "cheat day" to a "cheat meal" where once a week they eat a non-PV-approved meal and then are back on the wagon. But if you want a full day of unhampered gluttony, it's yours for the taking.

Here are my suggestions for a successful cheat day.

WRITE DOWN YOUR CRAVINGS. Throughout the week as you have cravings, write them down. This will help tame them. Just knowing as you write down "ice cream" or "oatmeal" that you'll

---

23 "Downregulation" refers to your metabolism slowing over time, often due to fasting or severe caloric restriction. Ferriss is suggesting that your metabolic rate will remain high due to the one-day-a-week cheat jumpstart.

have the opportunity in five days to eat as much of that item as you want goes a long way toward alleviating the urge to cave in and eat it now.

REVIEW YOUR LIST. On your cheat day, pull out your list of foods you wrote down during the week. Now—and this is key—don't discount any of them. If you want, you can eat your way line by line down the list. I'm serious. The only thing I ask of you is that you ask of yourself if you really want each item. Many times what was a hardcore craving in the moment turns into an "eh, I could live without that" food when you actually give yourself permission to eat it. Don't hold back though. If you really, really want french fries, don't try to make do with a lesser cheat like a piece of toast. It's called a cheat day for a reason. Eat the french fries so you stop obsessing about them and move on with life.

DRINK WATER. Drinking water helps flush out the system and fills you up. Sit down to whatever cheat foods and drinks you want, but also have a big glass of water by your side throughout the day to help negate the damage.

PUMP OUT A FEW BIG MUSCLE EXERCISES. Squats, wall push-ups, lunges, or even a short walk will help you continue to burn through calories and digest the food you're eating. Throw in ten deep squats and a few push-ups while you're baking the chocolate-chip cookies. C'mon…what other diet on the planet encourages that?

DON'T GET ON THE SCALE RIGHT AWAY. After experiencing my first cheat day on a Saturday, I nearly passed out Sunday morning when I stepped on the scale. I was up four pounds! Stupid, stupid, stupid cheat day! How could I have been suckered into believing this would work? I'm such an idiot…!

EASY DOES IT. Yes, your weight is going to be up after a cheat day, probably for the next several days after a cheat day. It will even out and, as you follow the PV diet for the remaining six days of the week, it will go down. So don't freak out about the scale.[24]

KEEP YOUR CARBS LOW. Ferriss advocates a cheat day for his Slow-Carb Diet, but remember that Slow-Carb does not allow for any starchy vegetables like sweet potatoes and turnips or any carb-laden sugars, like fruit. A Paleo Vegetarian diet does allow for these foods, so you may need to make modifications to either your weekly diet, by going lower in carbs, or to your cheat day, by not going quite as heavy on the carbs. Experiment and see what works for you.

MODERATE FOOD MANIA. Ferriss advocates all-out gluttony. And this is certainly an option. However, I'm going to advise a more moderate food mania. The first couple of times I did a cheat day, I made myself sick. Literally throwing up, lying on the couch, sick. That's what eating crap food will do to you. While an unpleasant sensation, it may be something each of us needs to go through. Friends who also do the cheat day note they had the same initial experience. I don't know if I got smarter or if my body adjusted, but over the course of about six weeks I stopped craving things like Little Debbie snacks and made my cheat days more about "healthier" foods in which I didn't indulge during the week. Fruit was a big one for me. Bananas with almond butter are my favorite snack on the planet, but I avoid bananas when I'm trying to lose weight because of all the sugar in them, and I can't keep almond butter in the house because it's like crack to me. So a cheat day for me usually holds a toasted gluten-free bagel with a sliced banana and almond butter. It's a cheat, but it's not like the half a Domino's pizza washed down with doughnut holes dipped in chocolate sauce I ate on my first cheat day. Other cheats for me may include a pasta dish, or I make an excellent Moroccan couscous dish with roasted

---

24 Actually, why do you even have a scale? Didn't I advise you to get rid of that thing. Ah-ha—caught you!

vegetables. Indulging in couscous may not sound like a cheat to some, but if it's a food you love and crave, it all tastes good.

But there's a caveat: Here's the deal. In order for cheat days to work, i.e., in order for you to be able to indulge in the crap foods, you must follow two rules, no exceptions:

A CHEAT DAY MUST BE PRECEDED BY A MINIMUM OF FIVE DAYS OF PV EATING. A once-a-week cheat day means just that. You can't have a cheat day on Saturday and then go out with friends on Tuesday and decide you'll make that a cheat day as well. The body needs time to reset before the next cheat day with at least five to six days of pure PV eating. And this brings us to rule number two…

NO CHEATING DURING THE WEEK. NONE. In order for cheat days to do what they're intended to do, i.e., reset your body, you must have an unblemished record of eating throughout the week. If you're sneaking a bite of bread here or a handful of chocolate there, your cheat day isn't a reset at all. And instead of helping you lose fat, you'll gain it. A perfect eating record during the week is the trade-off for your once-a-week free-for-all. Non-negotiable, folks.

The 80/20 Principle

Cheat days, as noted, come from the Slow-Carb Diet and aren't Paleo. Paleo, in its strictest sense, doesn't allow for cheats. Primal eating, however, and the world of Mark Sisson, advocates the use of the 80/20 principle[25] which, simply put, says if you eat right 80 percent of the time, it's okay to be a little looser with the rules the other 20 percent of the time. This isn't counting calories, and it differs from cheat days in several ways. First, an 80/20 plan

---

25 The 80/20 principle has nothing to do with calorie counting. It's based on a more subjective monitoring of whether or not your food intake matches a pure Paleo diet.

is not advocating a food free-for-all like the cheat day. Rather, it takes into account the practicalities of life and allows you to make adjustments as needed. There will be times when you're dining out or are with friends and there simply are no perfect PV options around. If that's the case, make the best of what's at hand and roll with it. Example: If it will break your mom's heart that you don't eat a slice of her home-baked apple pie, eat a slice of the pie. As long as you're sticking with the PV plan as a whole, a slip now and again is not going to send you into a tailspin.

Personally, I have a hard time following an 80/20 principle. That's because I, like most of us, tend to *underestimate* where that 20 percent line is. We eat some sandwich bread here, a bowl of cereal there, a taste of ice cream, a handful of peanuts, a bite of birthday cake, half a cookie…it all adds up and sooner than you think. For me, it's very easy for the 20 percent to slide into 30 percent to slide into 50 percent. Basically, I can't allow for cheat in moderation. If I had the sort of willpower that allowed me only the occasional indulgence, I wouldn't need to diet in the first place.

Still, especially if the PV plan you're following includes a good amount of fruit and starchy vegetables, an 80/20 path makes more sense than an all-out cheat day. Again, this may translate to a "cheat meal" once a week or simply eating clean PV all the time until those moments when there really isn't a good food choice available.

The idea behind both of these concepts is to recognize and allow for the fact that we're not perfect. Instead of fighting the imperfection, why not embrace it and make it work for you? Whether it's a cheat day or a 20 percent slip, take the time to enjoy and appreciate the food you eat—even the bad stuff. And, as a bonus, what I've found is that after a cheat day or cheat meal, my body craves healthy food. In fact, I am so eager to fill my body with healthy food that returning to a PV lifestyle for the next six days doesn't feel like a limitation. It feels like a gift.

Part II

Get in the Kitchen

Chapter 9

Embrace Your Inner Chef

Get ready to cook! And by that I mean that if you have less than a passing acquaintance with your stove and culinary utensils, it's time to stop by and reintroduce yourself. There is no shortchanging this—unless you want to eat cold salads 24/7, you *will* cook on the PV diet. And for those of you defying me, saying, "Heck yeah, I'll eat salad all day long. I LOVE me some salad!" you still have to chop and prep vegetables, so quit acting so smug. Bottom line, there is no Jenny Craig "pop-a-frozen-meal-in-the-microwave-and-dinner-is-ready" equivalent in the PV world.

Does this mean you need to be a gourmet chef? While I can't deny a week spent at Paris's Le Cordon Bleu would help, who has the time? No, it's not that bad. You can keep things simple with tips to help minimize time spent in the kitchen. But life will taste better if you're willing to spend maybe just a smidge more time in the kitchen than you currently do. Here are some of my best tips for getting in and out of the kitchen while having loads of great-tasting meals available at any time.

TIP #1: Organize your sh**. It's hard to be efficient in the kitchen when you can't find the sharp knife, your kids are using the cutting boards as the foundation for their Play-Doh castle, the Tupperware drawer looks like the cat ran through it, and the only measuring spoon available is the ⅛ teaspoon. Organize once, benefit forever. And remember to give yourself plenty of counter space. Tuck all the seldom-used or overly huge appliances away so your kitchen looks inviting for you to come in and cook.

TIP #2: Mark cooking time on your calendar. We're willing to schedule time for the "must do's" in our life like dental appointments and taking the dog to the groomer. Guess what? Your health just became a priority. And wishing you ate healthy food or wishing you stuck to your diet won't get you anywhere. Action is where it's at. If you love being in the kitchen, you may not need this. But if you know you're prone to putting off food prep, schedule a day and time, put it on the calendar, and honor it.

TIP #3: Meal planning. While you've got your calendar out, include some meal planning time in there. Frankly, I find this takes longer than the actual cooking. Remember though, you can keep it simple and eat the same meals over and over again. Those diet books that offer a different breakfast for every day of the week crack me up. Don't 90 percent of us pretty much eat the same thing for breakfast every day? But suddenly we're on a "diet" so we have to whip up fancy grain-free french toast before we leave for the office? I do best when I try one or two new recipes a week, max. On busy weeks I just eat the same three meals over and over again. Instead of being bored, I find it removes a source of stress. I know how to make this, it's fast, and it tastes decent. I'll save the "WOW!" meals for weekends or when I have the urge to cook.

TIP #4: Mise en place. The French term for "together in place," it means having everything assembled before you start cooking. Think of the chefs on TV shows who have all their ingredients chopped up in little bowls so they can just dump them in one at a time as the recipe calls for it. Sure, they have production assistants who prep all that, but that's what kids and significant others are for, right?

TIP #5: Recruit friends and family. If you're going to spend time in the kitchen, do what you can to make sure it's a joyous occasion—or at least doesn't suck. Listen to your favorite music, sip a glass of red wine, have your kids do their homework nearby, or ask a friend over and cook together. Call your mom and chat while you chop veggies. Catch up on your favorite podcast. The kitchen truly is the heart of your home. Make your time spent there something you look forward to.

TIP #6: Buy prechopped vegetables. I won't tell if you won't.

TIP #7: Pull out your slow cooker. Throw a bunch of veggies, spices, and marina sauce in your slow cooker in the morning, come home to the smell of heavenly slow-cooked vegetables ready to be added to a meal (throw it on top of baked spaghetti squash or cauliflower rice) at night.

TIP #8: Eat the skin. Forgo peeling. Vegetables like carrots, turnips, sweet potatoes, chopped eggplant, and beets can all be roasted skin-on. Just wash them well, stick them in the oven, and go.

TIP #9: Dice everything at once. I just love recipes that call for ¼ cup onion. So just what the frig am I supposed to do with the other peeled ¾ of it? Answer: Go ahead and dice it up too. The same goes for bell peppers, garlic, cabbage…you've got the knife and cutting board out, the countertop's already a mess, you're already invested in the cooking process. Just finish the job and put the extra chopped veggies in a resealable bag or storage container in the fridge. Now you're a step ahead of the game when you need chopped onion for a future recipe.

TIP #10: Portion out food as you cook it. As I finish cooking food, I'm divvying it up and storing it in containers for lunch and dinner. It saves the step of having to take one big container out of the fridge each morning to pack my lunch. Do this with nuts as well—put 10 to 12 almonds in a resalable bag and know that's your allotment for the day.

TIP #11: Bulk cooking. Here's how bulk cooking works.

- *Step 1: Pick Your Day.* Sundays work for me. I'm up early and don't have to be at the gym until 9 a.m. for my favorite BodyPump class, giving me 2 to 3 hours to get my cooking done.

- *Step 2: Prep Food for the Week.* I get the easy stuff out of the way first. I hard-boil about a dozen eggs, and while those are working, I start washing and prepping my vegetables. I chop the quick and easy stuff like the bell peppers and broccoli, and then while those are roasting, I prep the more time-consuming stuff like the brussels sprouts. Once I get in the groove, it's one big assembly line as food moves in and out of the oven.

- *Step 3: Roast/Boil/Slow-cook/Sauté.* Feel free to prepare your food any way you like. Me, I'm a roasting girl. Most bang for my buck, flavor wise, and I appreciate a cooking skill set that allows me to shove food into an oven and walk away for 30 minutes. Every Sunday morning is almost guaranteed to find me roasting broccoli, brussels sprouts, cauliflower, red/green/yellow/orange bell peppers, green beans (stop your howling that they're not Paleo; if they're in season, all the Paleo gods like Robb Wolf and Mark Sisson say it's okay), spaghetti squash, pattypan squash, and whatever vegetables are in my fridge at the end of the week that are about to go bad. (I usually have some mushrooms and sketchy grape tomatoes breathing their last breath that get thrown into the mix.) Other options include eggplant, kale, asparagus, broccolini, fennel, carrots…the list goes on. Don't be afraid to throw some garlic cloves in there either. Roasted garlic is divine, plus the smell keeps the vampires away. (Kidding.) I also typically make a simple egg fritatta (page 131) that I eat for either breakfast or lunch throughout the week. Go ahead and shred two heads of cauliflower so you have "rice" ready to be sautéed for the week. Also, wash your greens (kale, collards, Swiss chard) and go ahead and boil or sauté them.

Are you getting the idea? The secret is to double most any recipe and freeze the extra batch of soup or marinara or whatever it is you make. That way you have ready-to-go meals on the days or weeks you fall behind in your cooking.

My preference is to bulk cook once a week. If you have a large family, you may need to up it to twice a week. SUPER-prepared people cook once a month, but honestly, I don't think I have that much meal planning in me. My hat's off to you if you do.

If you're unaccustomed to bulk cooking, it can feel overwhelming at first. Give it a few tries, though, and see if, in the long run, it doesn't improve and open up significant windows of time in your life.

If It Tastes Good, Spit It Out

There is a group of retired gentlemen who, every day like clockwork, arrive at my gym at 5 a.m. They get their workout in and then hold court by the coffee machine for the next several hours. I adore this group and often head to the gym early so that I have enough time to sit and chat with them after I finish my workout.

During the process of writing this book, they kept tabs on my progress. One gentleman, a doctor, was and is less than taken with the idea of a Paleo Vegetarian diet, especially once I explained that meat, grains, beans, soy, dairy, and added sugars were on the banned foods list.

"So basically, if the food tastes good, they should spit it out," he said.

Everyone roared laughter, me included. I swore I would include that phrase somewhere in the book and so here it is.

Dr. Gloom aside, no, eating PV does *not* mean you only get to eat bland food. So let's dig in. We've spent enough time talking about what you're not going to eat on this diet. It's time to switch gears and talk about the foods that will actually fill your plate.

Include at Least Two or Three of These Foods in Every Meal

The challenge for PVers is getting enough protein and omega-3s in your diet. The list below is by no means a comprehensive one of foods you can eat. However, the foods on this list are high in either healthy fat, protein, or omega-3s. For that reason, aim to include as many and as much of these foods in your diet as possible.

- Fish and seafood (if a part of your diet)
- Whole eggs (pasture-raised preferred)
- Flax and chia seeds
- Hemp seed
- Olive oil

- Nuts, especially walnuts (pecans and pine nuts as well)
- Leafy greens—kale, spinach, collards, Swiss chard, mustard greens, etc.
- Cabbage
- Broccoli
- Avocados (limit to one per day if trying to lose weight)
- Brussels sprouts
- Seaweed—kelp and spirulina
- Berries
- Potatoes (for athletes or after hard workouts)

One Last Word about Beans

We've already touched on the topic of including beans in your diet, but as we move into the recipe section, it bears repeating.

Once again, beans are unequivocally *not* Paleo. As covered in the introductory section of this book, beans (or legumes) contain phytic acid. Phytic acid prevents the body's absorption of nutrients. Not a huge problem if eaten in small amounts, but a definite challenge when consumed in large quantity. Beans are also carbohydrate-dense, which can make losing weight even more of a challenge if your diet is high in beans.

So where's the debate? The issue is I'm going to toss you a curve ball and say that the *occasional* use of beans in your diet is okay. There are, in fact, a number of recipes just ahead that contain beans—chilis and pizza crusts and a lentil soup. Why?

Mainly because beans are an easy source of protein. Paleoists note that there are better sources of protein, ones that don't contain phytic acid, and that's true—if you eat meat and animal fats. Paleo Vegetarians don't, and so your protein sources are much more limited. For that reason, I'm not above your tossing the occasional handful of beans into your salads or using them to make a substitute pizza crust (see pages 151 and 153). I don't recommend you make beans a staple of every meal, but ½ cup of beans a day probably isn't going to ruin your world.

Green beans are the exception. There are the die-hard Paleo purists who insist that since green beans are pods, they count as beans and are therefore unacceptable on the Paleo diet. However, the Paleo and Primal gurus Robb Wolf and Mark Sisson both agree that eating green beans in-season is Paleo acceptable. So long as they remain a side dish and not a diet staple, you're safe enjoying them a couple of times a week as a side item or tossed into a stir-fry, soup, or stew.

While we're on the topic, the same can be said for snow peas. You don't want to gorge on them, but an occasional helping isn't going to wreck your diet. I have a favorite frozen vegetable medley mix I buy each week that contains broccoli, red peppers, cauliflower, and probably six snow pea pods in the entire 12-ounce bag. I could pick them out but then I remember, "oh yeah, I have a life"—and I eat them and move on.

So let's get to it. The recipes. What follows are but a smattering of the wide array of foods available to you. I've included examples of strict PV items such as a delicious roasted cabbage soup and breakfast (or dinner!) quiche. There are also some bean-infused soups and chilies that can be eaten in moderation to add protein to your diet and may be especially important for high-intensity PV athletes to use for fuel and recovery. There are also some fun PV sweets like a pumpkin streusel and organic coconut chocolate balls. These are more special-occasion treats, but I wanted to show you that you can still have healthy PV-friendly foods *without* having to wait for a cheat day.

I've also included a number of what I consider PV basics: cauliflower rice and mashed potatoes, Paleo bread, and simple Paleo pancakes.

Almost all of these recipes have been modified or inspired by what were once non-PV-friendly recipes. A deletion of corn here, an insertion of kale there, and voilá! PV deliciousness on a plate.

I encourage you to peruse Paleo and vegetarian websites to come up with your own PV culinary inspirations. But don't feel you need to cook up a storm. The majority of your meals can remain quite simple: roasted vegetables doused in coconut or olive oil, big, fresh leafy-green salads, soft scrambled eggs served with slices of tender avocado.

Who's ready to eat?

How the Recipes Are Organized

A quick browse of the recipes in the following chapters will reveal a lack of standard recipe book classifications, like "Breakfast," "Lunch," "Dinner," and "Snacks." That's because I stand by my mantra that any food can be delicious and filling eaten at any time. Pizza for breakfast and "Breakfast Quiche" for dinner? You bet. Therefore, I've arranged recipes by type, such as "Egg Dishes" and "Salads, Soups, and Greens." There's also a "Just Try It" section that contains recipes that may be outside the norm *or* require more prep work than the rest. You may not make these every week, but they're still delicious and filling, and you know what? You should try them!

Chapter 10

Egg Dishes

FALL FRITTATA

I was honored to perform the marriage ceremony for my friends Nathan and Katie. Both runners, both foodies, their home is filled not only with love, but with the sweet and savory smells of the delectable dishes they create daily. You can read more about the meals they create at Katie's blog, LivingTheKatieWay.com. Meanwhile, the savory flavors of this frittata are perfect for a fall meal (or any time of year!) when paired with a salad of arugula and sliced almonds tossed with lemon juice and extra virgin olive oil. SERVES 4

1 teaspoon coconut oil (more if not using a nonstick or cast-iron pan)

1 medium onion, sliced

1 bulb fennel, sliced

1 to 2 cloves garlic, minced

7 pasture-raised eggs

2 tablespoons vegetable broth or water

1 teaspoon salt

10 to 12 fresh sage leaves

Tip: Use a well-seasoned cast-iron skillet to make a frittata without leaving a mess behind!

1. Preheat the oven's broiler.

2. Heat the coconut oil in a medium oven-safe pan over low heat.

3. Add the onion and cook for about 5 minutes, until the onion begins to soften.

4. Add the fennel and garlic. Continue to cook over low heat, stirring occasionally, until the onion begins to caramelize.

5. In a medium bowl, whisk the eggs then combine them with the broth and salt.

6. As the onions begin to caramelize, spread the onion, fennel and garlic evenly across the bottom of the pan.

7. Gently pour the egg mixture over the vegetables, then scatter sage leaves across the pan.

8. Cook on the stovetop over low heat, using a spatula to loosen the egg from the sides of the pan, until the sides begin to look set, about 2 to 3 minutes.

9. Place the pan under the broiler and broil until the egg is set, about 5 minutes.

SERVING IDEAS

- Up the nutrient level by adding fresh spinach or any leafy green.
- Change up the vegetables—red bell peppers, mushrooms, asparagus, eggplant…Seriously, what doesn't go with egg?
- Add ¼ to ½ cup of well-rinsed black beans for a protein boost.
- Eat for breakfast, lunch, dinner, or a snack.
- If you eat fish, pair this with smoked salmon or any type of baked fish for a protein-packed meal.

BREAKFAST QUICHE

This is a great staple to have in the refrigerator when you're in a rush.
It freezes well in individual serving sizes. SERVES 4

8 pasture-raised eggs
1 teaspoon salt
2 teaspoons pepper
½ large onion, diced

2 medium zucchini, chopped
1 medium head broccoli,
   chopped

1. Preheat oven to 350°F.

2. Spray an 8 x 8-inch square pan or 9-inch pie dish with coconut oil or olive oil cooking spray.

3. In a medium bowl, whisk the eggs, salt, and pepper.

4. Stir in the chopped vegetables and stir to combine.

5. Pour the contents of the bowl into the baking dish and bake for 25 to 30 minutes, or until the eggs are set. Remove from the heat and let sit for 5 minutes before serving.

SERVING IDEAS

- Pour the quiche into a sprayed muffin pan for easy individual servings.

- Have your way with vegetables. Try a spinach-asparagus combo, a mushroom-red pepper quiche, or a Mexican-inspired tomato and black olive creation.

- Quiche pairs beautifully with a salad or a grilled portobello mushroom for a light yet filling meal.

- Quiche and half a baked sweet potato are an excellent recovery meal after a hard cardio session.

VEGGIE-EGG MUFFINS

I love these muffins as a quick go-to snack. They're also ideal food-on-the-go. Double the recipe and freeze the muffins and you'll have protein goodness at your fingertips any time you need it. Frozen spinach and vegetables work great here. Just thaw them out first. For the spinach, be sure to wring out excess water or else the muffins will be gloppy. MAKES 12 MUFFINS OR 6 SERVINGS

8 pasture-raised eggs
2 cups diced veggies of
your choice (red or green
pepper, yellow or red onion,
mushrooms, asparagus,
broccoli, spinach, kale, etc.

¼ teaspoon salt (optional)
¼ teaspoon black pepper
1 to 2 tablespoons water

1. Preheat the oven to 350°F.

2. Spray a muffin pan with coconut or olive oil cooking spray.

3. In a medium bowl, whisk the eggs, then add in all the vegetables and the salt, pepper, and water. Stir to make sure all vegetables are evenly coated. It's okay to add a little more water if the mixture seems too thick or not liquid enough to coat all the vegetables.

4. Fill each muffin cup three-quarters full with the egg-veggie mixture.

5. Bake for about 20 minutes, until a toothpick inserted into the center of a muffin comes out clean.

SERVING IDEAS

- Serve between halves of a red bell pepper with baby spinach for a lunchtime sandwich.

- Spice the muffins up with a dash of hot sauce or some chilies added in before baking.

- Make Mediterranean-inspired muffins with sun-dried tomatoes, black olives, and a tiny bit of feta cheese.

Chapter 11

Salads, Soups, and Greens

COLLARD WRAPS WITH RAW CURRIED CARROT PÂTÉ

Ricki Heller (RickiHeller.com) is a cookbook author, professional recipe developer, holistic nutritionist, and anti-candida crusader. This recipe is the ideal PV recipe, as it's low-glycemic and high in protein. It's even vegan-friendly. Ricki says, "this pâté is perfect over crackers, in wraps, or as a light meal alongside a salad. Apart from soaking the seeds, it comes together in a snap." SERVES 6 TO 8 AS AN APPETIZER, 3 OR 4 AS A MAIN DISH

1 cup raw sunflower seeds, soaked in room temperature water for 2 hours (or up to overnight, covered in the refrigerator)

1 large carrot, peeled and cut in chunks

1 clove garlic, chopped

½-inch round fresh peeled ginger, minced (about 2 teaspoons)

2 teaspoons white or light miso

½ teaspoon curry powder

½ to 1 teaspoon sriracha (or use a generous pinch of cayenne pepper)

½ teaspoon coconut aminos

1 tablespoon freshly squeezed lemon juice

sea salt, to taste

4 large collard leaves, halved and ribs removed (i.e., 8 halves once cut)

Add-ins (choose 3 to 5, to your taste): sprouts, grape tomatoes, grated carrot, sauerkraut, sliced green onion, avocado, hummus, or other veggies of choice, chopped

1. Place all the ingredients except the collard leaves and add-ins in the bowl of a food processor and process until almost smooth, scraping the sides of the bowl as needed.

2. To assemble the rolls, lay out the collard leaves (they will be half-leaves once the midrib is removed) on a flat surface. Spread each half with about one-eighth of the pâté, then line up 3 to 5 of the add-ins on one end of the leaf. Starting at the end with the add-ins, roll up the leaf as you would sushi. Cut into four smaller rolls for appetizers, or in half for a main course. Serve immediately.

If you have extra pâté, it can be stored, covered, in the refrigerator for up to 5 days.

SERVING IDEAS

- Use your own mixes of ingredients to adapt the recipe to your own tastes.

ROASTED CAULIFLOWER SOUP

This recipe was submitted by my good friend and fellow pet lover Sena Crutchley. Sena is a long-time vegetarian and the person who taught me to make homemade seiten. Seiten's not on the PV diet, but being a stellar cook, Sena's always up for a recipe challenge. Thanks Sena, for the soup! SERVES 6

1 head cauliflower, cut into bite-size florets

2 tablespoons olive oil, divided

2 teaspoons salt, divided

1 cup soaked cashews (*soak the cashews overnight or for at least a couple of hours in water)

7 cups flax milk (or other nondairy milk like almond or coconut), divided

½ sweet onion, chopped

½ teaspoon garam masala

2 cloves garlic, crushed

1 teaspoon ground cumin

½ teaspoon ground turmeric

½ teaspoon ground coriander

½ cup shelled and unsalted pistachios

1. Preheat the oven to 400°F.

2. Toss the cauliflower in a medium bowl with 1 tablespoon olive oil and 1 teaspoon of salt. Add more oil if the cauliflower isn't well coated. Roast the cauliflower on a baking sheet in the oven for 30 minutes.

3. While the cauliflower is roasting, blend the drained cashews with 1 cup of the flax milk until very smooth.

4. Warm the remaining 1 tablespoon olive oil in a medium pan over medium heat. Add the onion and sauté until transparent but not brown, about 6 to 8 minutes.

5. In large pot, combine the remaining 6 cups of flax milk with the blended cashews, sautéed onions, garam masala, garlic, cumin, turmeric, coriander, and the remaining salt. Heat over medium-high heat and bring to a gentle rolling boil. Reduce the heat and let simmer for 5 minutes.

6. Puree the roasted cauliflower and then stir into the pot with the milk mixture.

7. Garnish each serving with pistachios.

SERVING IDEAS

- Fresh greens (kale, mustard greens, collards, spinach, etc.) stirred into the soup taste delicious and add a power boost.

- Serve with a side salad for a warm and satisfying meal.

- Soup for breakfast? Yes! This soup can easily take the place of your morning oatmeal.

SAVORY GREEN STUFFING

This is a modified version of a recipe I found in a book called 366 Healthful Ways to Cook Leafy Greens. *Don't be shy about playing with a variation of herbs and spices to lend the dish a different taste. This dish reheats well, which makes it useful as a post-workout recovery food as well.* SERVES 4 AS A SIDE DISH, 2 AS A MAIN DISH

1 tablespoon olive oil or coconut oil
½ cup yellow onion, chopped
12 ounces frozen greens (spinach, kale, collards, mustard greens, etc.), thawed, liquid reserved

1 cup almond meal
½ cup vegetable broth
1 pasture-raised egg
1 teaspoon dried basil
salt and pepper

1. Preheat the oven to 375°F. Spray an 8 x 8-inch baking dish with coconut oil cooking spray and set aside.

2. Heat the oil over medium heat in a medium pan and add the chopped onion. Sauté until translucent, about 5 to 7 minutes, and remove from heat.

3. In a large bowl, mix together the onions and all the remaining ingredients (including the juice from thawed greens), making sure all ingredients are well coated.

4. Pour the mixture into the baking pan. Cover with foil and bake for 15 minutes.

5. Remove the foil and bake another 5 to 10 minutes, until the mixture is heated through.

SERVING IDEAS

- Eat as a side dish or use as a stuffing for red bell pepper sandwiches or in "deviled" hard-boiled eggs.

- Serve on top of mixed greens or shredded cabbage.

- Toss a handful of walnuts on top for extra crunch.

- Serve with a side of fried or scrambled eggs.

- Serve inside a roasted sweet potato for a filling meal.

ROASTED CABBAGE SOUP

Another culinary masterpiece from Nathan and Katie at LivingTheKatieWay.com. Per Katie, "Roasting the cabbage in this recipe before placing it into the soup makes for a richer eating experience!" MAKES ABOUT 8 CUPS OR 3 TO 5 SERVINGS

1 head red or green cabbage (3 to 4 pounds), sliced thinly

4 tablespoons extra-virgin olive oil, divided

2 teaspoons salt, divided

4 carrots, peeled and diced

1 large sweet onion, diced

1 pound turnips, peeled and chopped

4 cups vegetable broth

2 to 4 cups water

1. Preheat the oven to 375°F.

2. Toss the cabbage with 3 tablespoons of olive oil and 1 teaspoon of salt until well-coated, then spread evenly on a large baking sheet.

3. Bake the cabbage for 45 to 60 minutes, turning the cabbage every 15 minutes until it's browned in spots. Remove from the oven and set aside.

4. While the cabbage is roasting, in a large pan, sauté the carrots and onion with the remaining 1 tablespoon of olive oil and 1 teaspoon of salt over low heat until the carrot begins to soften and the onion is partially translucent.

5. Add the cabbage and turnips and stir well. Add the vegetable broth and enough water to cover all the vegetables.

6. Bring to a boil, then reduce the heat to low and cover.

7. Stir occasionally and cook for about 30 minutes, or until all the vegetables are tender. Add more water as needed to keep vegetables covered.

SERVING IDEAS

- If you eat seafood, add a handful of shrimp for a power boost.

- This is great to eat an hour or two before a workout.

- Double the recipe and freeze it for some quick meals on the go.

MUSHROOM, SQUASH, AND KALE SALAD

This is one of those recipes that, upon hearing the name, makes meat lovers wrinkle their noses at the "rabbit food" we call a main meal. That is, until they taste it. Personally, I refuse them second servings until they formally apologize for prejudging. SERVES 2 AS A MAIN DISH

1 tablespoon coconut oil or olive oil

½ cup minced yellow onion

1 cup chopped mushrooms of any variety

1 bunch kale, washed and torn into pieces

1 cup cooked and cubed butternut squash (page 171)

¼ cup feta cheese (optional)

1. Heat the oil in a large pan over medium heat.

2. Sauté the onions and mushrooms for a few minutes, and then add the kale. Continue sautéing until the onions are tender, about 5 to 7 minutes.

3. Add the cooked squash and stir to combine.

4. Top with feta.

SERVING IDEAS

- It's hard to improve on perfection, and this meal is up there. But everything goes with kale, so substitute or add in any veggies of your choice.

- If you eat seafood, this is a great side dish alongside fish or shrimp.

- Serve over Basic Cauliflower Rice (page 148).

BIG-ASS SALAD

Most people have their own version of a Big-Ass Salad. My typical ingredients are, well, pretty much anything leftover I'm looking to get rid of. I start with a base of baby spinach then raid the fridge and add on from there. SERVES 1 TO 12 DEPENDING ON HOW MUCH YOU MAKE!

Base

baby spinach and/or chopped kale (cooked or uncooked)

Toppings—Any Combination of

roasted brussels sprouts

roasted cauliflower

roasted red peppers

roasted or raw broccoli

roasted asparagus

sautéed mushrooms

artichoke hearts, canned, in water

sliced zucchini and/or yellow squash

handful of olives (kalamata, black, green, etc.)

Optional Ingredients

handful of nuts (walnuts, almonds, sunflower seeds, etc.)

grated carrots

few slices mandarin oranges

sliced cucumber

½ avocado, sliced

Optional Proteins

½ cup beans (black, pinto, or chickpeas)

sliced hard-boiled pasture-raised egg

salmon

tuna

shrimp

sardines

Dressing

olive oil, balsamic vinegar, pepper to taste

1. Pull out a massive plate or bowl. Pile on ingredients. Take a deep breath. Dig in and enjoy.

SERVING IDEAS

• Add some toasted Basic Cauliflower Rice (page 148).

• If you're eating fruit, toss in a handful of grapes or a few slices of green or red apple.

• Scoop a handful of the salad inside half a red bell pepper.

Chapter 12

Classic Standbys

B.S. BURGERS

The real name for this recipe is "Brussels Sprouts Burgers" and is based on a recipe I found on http://cavemanketo.com/brussel-sprout-burgers. However, around our house it became known as the "B.S. Burger" because the first time I ever made it, I was in full-blown vegetarian mode. When my meat-eating husband called and asked what was for dinner and I said, "Burgers," he responded with a knee-jerk, "Bullsh**!"

The name aside, these burgers are chock-full of protein and are delicious on their own, on top of Paleo Bread (page 155), or I like them for breakfast or dinner with a fried egg on top! SERVES 2 TO 4

16 ounces Cashew Cheese
  (page 145)
1 (16-ounce) bag brussels
  sprouts (about 25)
¼ cup diced green onion,
  white and green parts

⅓ cup almond flour
10 ounces goat cheese
  (optional)
3 pasture-raised eggs
4 tablespoons coconut oil
salt and pepper

1. Prepare the Cashew Cheese. (The cheese can be made ahead and will keep in the fridge for up to a week.)

2. Rinse the brussels sprouts under cool water then shred them. Use a food processor to save time or, if you're hardcore, grate them by hand.

3. Combine the green onion, Cashew Cheese, and almond floor in a small bowl, then add to the shredded brussels sprouts. Crumble in the goat cheese. Season with salt and pepper to taste.

4. Whisk the eggs and add to the brussels sprouts, mixing well to coat all the pieces. Use a fork to mash the goat cheese in, if using. The mixture should be thick and sticky at this point.

5. Divide the mixture into even-sized patties.

6. Melt the coconut oil in a skillet over medium-high heat, then add the "burger" patties.

7. Cook on each side until crisp, about 1 to 3 minutes per side.

SERVING IDEAS

- Use B.S. Burgers as "bread" to hold a grilled portobello mushroom and roasted red peppers.

- Turn the burgers into breakfast (or dinner!) with the addition of a fried egg.

- Create a B.S. Burger Tower: layer one burger, one layer of vegetables, one burger, one layer of goat cheese, one burger, another layer of vegetables, etc. Messy? Yes. But fun! And oh-so filling.

CASHEW CHEESE

Cashew cheese? Gesundheit! (I crack myself up…) MAKES ENOUGH FOR 1 RECIPE OF B.S. BURGERS (PAGE 143), PLUS A LITTLE EXTRA

1 pound cashews
1 to 2 lemons (enough for ½ cup lemon juice)
2 tablespoons coconut oil

1 to 2 cloves garlic or ½ teaspoon garlic powder (optional)
sea salt and pepper, to taste

1. Pour the cashews in a large bowl, cover with water, and let them sit overnight. In the morning, drain them and place in a food processor.

2. Process the cashews. Once they have broken down a bit, add the remaining ingredients. You may need to add a little water as you go along, but *add slowly*. The ingredients will become creamier the longer you process them—don't rush.

SERVING IDEAS

- Use as a dip for vegetables.

- Use as a condiment in place of mayonnaise. I like to cut a red pepper in half, smear with a tablespoon of cashew cheese, and stuff with sprouts and vegetables for a ready-made sandwich.

- Impress guests: Stuff pitted medjool dates with cashew cheese and top with chopped almonds or fruit.

ZIPPY ZUCCHINI FRIES

Sometimes you just need fries. 'Nuff said. SERVES 2

1 pasture-raised egg
¼ teaspoon water
1 large zucchini

½ cup almond meal
salt and pepper

1. Preheat the oven to 425°F. Spray a baking sheet with coconut oil cooking spray.

2. Whisk the egg with the water.

3. Slice zucchini into french fry–like strips. Dip each strip in the egg, then roll in the almond meal and place on the baking sheet.

4. Bake for about 30 minutes, until fries are slightly browned.

5. Remove from oven. Add salt and pepper to taste.

SERVING IDEAS

- You can substitute most any vegetable to add some crispness to your meals.

- Eat them with a side of spicy mustard.

PV PANCAKES

Pancakes seem to be the number one thing people miss most on a Paleo diet. For that reason, there are a huge number of Paleo pancake recipes out there that use everything from pumpkin to coconut to bananas. I'm including a banana recipe below because, with three ingredients, it just doesn't get any easier. This makes a great pre- or post-workout snack. SERVES 1

1 banana   ½ teaspoon cinnamon
1 pasture-raised egg

1. Mash the banana with a fork or food processor, then beat in the egg.

2. Add the cinnamon and give a quick stir.

3. Heat a nonstick[26] frying pan coated in coconut oil cooking spray over medium heat. Pour in 2 to 3 small pancake shapes.

4. Once bubbles appear on the surface of each pancake, flip and cook on the second side until done.

SERVING IDEAS

• Add a teaspoon of shredded coconut or a small handful of blueberries to the batter.

• Add a dash of vanilla extract to the batter.

• Add ¼ cup of pumpkin puree and also top with a bit of the puree to bring out the flavor.

• Top with almond butter.

• Slide a fried egg in between two pancakes for a power meal.

---

26 Trust me on this. Go with nonstick. The banana mixture gets sticky on a regular pan, even when sprayed. If using a regular pan, add a little fat in there, like some butter or coconut oil.

BASIC CAULIFLOWER RICE

While not quite as dead-on in taste to white rice as cauliflower mashed potatoes are to real potatoes, this recipe is still a game changer. The recipe below is pretty bland, which is fine if you're just using it as a base to smother in savory vegetables and sauces. However, if you want to actually serve "rice" as a side dish, I'd suggest amping up the taste with one of the serving ideas listed with the recipe. MAKES APPROXIMATELY 2 CUPS

1 head cauliflower

1 onion, finely chopped

2 tablespoons ghee or coconut oil

salt and pepper

1. Chop the cauliflower into chunks. Use a food processor or hand grater to grate the cauliflower into a rice-like consistency.

2. Melt the ghee or coconut oil in a pan over medium heat.

3. Add the onion and sauté until softened, about 5 minutes.

4. Add the cauliflower and mix well with the onion and fat.

5. You can either cover the pan for 5 to 10 minutes to cook the cauliflower or treat it like a stir-fry and turn the heat up a bit, stirring the cauliflower frequently until it just starts to brown. Don't overcook.

6. Season with salt and pepper to taste, and serve.

A WORD ABOUT CAULIFLOWER

I can't emphasize enough the importance cauliflower will take on in your life. Delicious raw or roasted, cauliflower can be transformed into mashed potatoes or rice, and is neutral enough to take on any flavor to give your meals an added boost. Enjoy the recipes below and feel free to add more spices to your liking.

SERVING IDEAS

- Add different spices for different flavors: lime/cilantro; curry/cinnamon/cardamom for Indian flavor; taco seasoning mix/diced tomatoes in juice/green chilies for Mexican flair; etc.
- Use as a base for vegetable stir-fries.
- Stir into soups and stews.
- Serve under two fried eggs for a new twist on breakfast.
- Serve under fish, portobello mushrooms, or as a savory side dish.

"YOU WON'T BELIEVE THEY'RE NOT MASHED POTATOES" MASHED POTATOES

You. Must. Try. These. I have served these mashed "potatoes" time and again, never revealing until after the first bite has been taken that they're actually just pureed cauliflower. It's like a party trick—people lose their minds. For once, this isn't a "substitute" food, as the taste and texture is dead-on to "real" mashed potatoes. MAKES 2 LARGE SERVINGS

1 head fresh cauliflower or 1 (12-ounce) bag frozen cauliflower

2 tablespoons butter or ghee, or more
salt and pepper

Tip: You can substitute turnips for the same effect. Just boil turnips until soft (check with a fork) then follow the same instructions below.

1. If using fresh cauliflower, chop into large chunks.

2. Bring a pot of water to a boil.

3. Add the fresh or frozen cauliflower and return the water to a boil. Boil for about 5 minutes, until the cauliflower has softened.

4. Place the cauliflower in a food processor along with butter, salt, and pepper as desired. Puree until combined.

SERVING IDEAS

- Use the above recipe as a base and play with flavors. Add chives and garlic. Experiment with curry. Go for a smoky taste with roasted red peppers and adobo sauce.

- Serve alongside grilled portobello mushrooms for a "steak and potatoes" dinner.

- Smother the potatoes in mushrooms and Paleo gravy.

- Use the cauliflower as a topping on a vegetable potpie. (Remember to use a Paleo crust!)

CAULIFLOWER CRUST

This recipe is a combination of a number of cauliflower recipes I've tried. Many suggest adding spices or cheese to the mix, but I prefer this simple recipe as I really use my crust less for taste and more as a vehicle to hold my other ingredients. Feel free to experiment to get the crust to your liking. MAKES 1 (10 TO 12-INCH) PIZZA CRUST

½ head cauliflower, shredded (use either a hand grater or a food processor)
1 pasture-raised egg

organic, low-sugar tomato sauce
your favorite pizza toppings

1. Preheat the oven to 450°F.

2. Microwave the shredded cauliflower in a microwave-safe bowl until tender, about 3 minutes. Use your hands to wring out excess water (careful!—it will be hot) and allow to cool. Don't skip the cooldown or you'll cook the egg when you add it!

3. Whisk the egg in a small bowl. *Slowly* combine the egg with the cauliflower—you don't want the mixture overly soggy. It's okay if you don't use the whole egg. Mix well.

4. Spray a baking sheet with coconut oil cooking spray. Use your hands to form the egg and cauliflower mixture into a pizza shape in the center of the tray. Make the crust as thin or thick as you desire. If the mixture is goopy, add more cauliflower; too dry, add more egg.

PIZZA! PIZZA!

I will not live in a world without pizza. Luckily, I don't have to. Below are two different pizza crust recipes—one made from cauliflower and one from a white bean paste. Beans aren't Paleo, so consider this crust an occasional hack for times when you need the added protein. By the way, a small slice of pizza makes a great pre- or post-workout snack!

5. Slide into the oven and bake for 20 minutes, until slightly browned, flipping once halfway through.

6. Remove from the oven. Spread with tomato sauce and your favorite toppings. Cook under the broiler for 5 minutes or place back in oven at 400°F for about 10 to 12 minutes.

SERVING IDEAS

- Toss on handfuls of spinach and kale for added nutritional value.

- Instead of pizza, cut the crust into strips and use as dipping sticks in marinara sauce or Cashew Cheese (page 145).

- Roll the crust out super thin, brush with olive oil, and dust with sea salt, pepper, and/or grated Parmesan cheese. Break apart after baking to create crackerlike snacks.

- Use the crust as sandwich bread—layer in your favorite veggies like kale, Portobello mushrooms, sprouts, etc.

WHITE BEAN CRUST

Inspired by "My Favorite Slow-Carb Pizza Recipe" at http://www. findingmyfitness.com/2012/03/my-favorite-slow-carb-pizza-recipe, you may want to eat these yummy pizzas in the privacy of your home. The first time I took leftovers into my office for lunch, I spent 20 minutes fending off, "But you don't eat bread!" exclamations as I dug in. MAKES 1 (8 X 8-INCH) PIZZA CRUST

1 teaspoon olive oil

2 cups navy or cannellini beans, cooked or canned

½ teaspoon garlic salt (optional)

1 teaspoon Italian seasoning

1 pasture-raised egg

tomato sauce and other favorite pizza toppings

1. Preheat the oven to 375°F. Spray a baking sheet or 8 x 8-inch baking pan with olive oil or coconut oil cooking spray.

2. Heat the olive oil in small pan over medium-high heat. Add the beans and stir until they begin to break and fall apart, usually 5 to 7 minutes. (Alternatively, you can microwave the beans, covered with a bit of water, until they turn soft.)

3. Transfer the beans to a small bowl and mash them with a fork. Add the garlic salt, if using, and Italian seasoning and combine well.

4. Once the beans cool, whisk the egg and add it to the bean mix. Form into a pizza shape on the baking sheet or spread in the baking pan.

5. Bake the crust until firm, about 15 minutes.

6. Remove from oven, spread with tomato sauce and your favorite toppings. Place under the broiler for 5 minutes, or place back in the oven at 400°F for 10 to 12 minutes.

SERVING IDEAS

• See Cauliflower Crust recipe serving ideas (page 152).

SUPER-DUPER SPAGHETTI SQUASH

Who needs a plate of thick, doughy, food-coma-inducing pasta when a lighter, delicious alternative is so readily available? A big plate of spaghetti squash makes a filling meal, but don't forget about it as a side item to round out a lunch or breakfast. SERVES 4

1 spaghetti squash, any size   salt and pepper
½ cup water

1. Preheat the oven to 350°F.

2. Use a large knife to cut the squash in half lengthwise, and scrape out the seeds.

3. Place the squash face-down in a deep, rimmed baking dish with the water.

4. Bake for about 1 hour. The squash is done when you can pierce the skin with a fork. Be careful not to overcook, as the squash will turn mushy.

5. Remove the squash and use a large fork to scrape out the insides into long strings. Add salt and pepper to taste.

SERVING IDEAS

- Top with marinara sauce and your favorite veggies.

- Toss lightly with olive oil, fresh herbs, and sun-dried tomatoes.

- Use the squash as a base in a dish like Pad Thai.

- Toss with chopped kale, mushrooms, and artichoke hearts.

- Sauté your favorite vegetables in some spices, whisk an egg, add some diced tomatoes, add in the spaghetti squash, put all the ingredients into a casserole dish, and bake for an additional 30 to 40 minutes at 350°F until golden brown on top.

- This is great paired with Stuffed Eggplant (page 164).

- Add beans or lentils to any of the above for added protein.

PALEO BREAD

I'll be honest. I made my own Paleo bread a couple of times, but my heart wasn't in it. I now buy my bread in bulk from JulianBakery.com and store it in the freezer, taking out a half loaf at a time to portion throughout the week. Again, be cautious you don't become overly dependent on premade Paleo products, choosing fresh, whole foods instead. But for me, one piece of toast a day spread with avocado makes me happy. And if you're inclined to make your own bread, this is a delicious recipe.

Below is a basic bread recipe. I will say that Paleo breads don't quite match up to regular breads in terms of texture. I've had more than one piece crumble apart on me in the toaster. Luckily, I'm not above turning the toaster upside down and banging on it to capture toast crumbs. MAKES 1 LOAF

6 pasture-raised eggs
½ cup melted butter, ghee, or
   coconut oil
¼ cup honey
¼ cup ground golden flax
   seed

½ cup almond butter
½ teaspoon sea salt
½ teaspoon baking soda
¾ cup coconut or almond
   flour

1. Preheat the oven to 350°F. Use coconut oil to grease a 9 x 5-inch loaf pan or line it with parchment paper.

2. Place all the ingredients in a large bowl or food processor and blend until smooth.

3. Pour the mixture into a prepared 9 x 5 loaf pan.

4. Bake for about 40 minutes, until an inserted toothpick comes out clean.

5. The bread will keep in the fridge, wrapped in plastic wrap, for 3 to 7 days or in the freezer for one month.

SERVING IDEAS

- It's bread! Do you really need serving ideas?

Chapter 13

Just Try It

NUTTY OLIVE PÂTÉ

Another recipe from my friend Sena, this one taking advantage of the nutritional combination of mushrooms, walnuts, and flax seed. This is an elegant "share with friends" dish, especially those friends who are convinced you are wilting away, gnawing on tasteless, droopy carrot tops for the majority of your meals. SERVES 4 AS AN APPETIZER

1 tablespoon olive oil
½ cup finely chopped sweet
   onion
2 cups button or cremini
   mushrooms
1 (6-ounce) can black pitted
   olives

½ cup finely chopped walnuts
1 tablespoon ground flax seed
¼ teaspoon salt
¼ teaspoon garlic powder
⅛ teaspoon black pepper

1. Preheat the oven to 350°F.

2. Warm the olive oil in a small pan over low heat, add the onion, and sauté until the onion is browned and beginning to caramelize.

3. While the onion is sautéing, mince the mushrooms and olives in a food processor or chopper.

4. Combine the mushrooms, olives, walnuts, flax seed, salt, garlic powder, and black pepper in a medium bowl. Add the onions to the mixture and again thoroughly mix. Feel free to add other flavors according to personal taste. For example, this pâté is delicious with 1 tablespoon of diced roasted red peppers mixed into it.

5. Scoop the mixture into mini rectangular loaf pans and press firmly. The size of the pans will determine how many will be needed.

5. Bake uncovered for 30 minutes.

6. Chill in the refrigerator overnight. Remove from the pan before serving.

SERVING IDEAS

- Serve with crudité, which is a fancy way of saying sliced or whole raw vegetables.
- Take breakfast from ho-hum to *"Damn!"* by adding pâté as a side to a broccoli and red pepper omelet.
- Serve with a side of fruit.
- Stuff the pâté into vegetables such as a whole red pepper or tomato or on top of celery.
- Use as a tantalizing topper on salads.

GREEN MOUNTAIN GRINGO VEGETARIAN CHILI

This chili recipe from friend and chef extraordinaire Michael O'Donnell, Corporate Executive Chef for the TW Garner Food Company, takes some effort but I promise you, the payoff is more than worth it. Hearty, flavorful, spicy, and very delicious. YUM.

MAKES 6 TO 8 SERVINGS

4 to 5 tablespoons olive oil

1 red onion, diced

10 large cloves garlic, sliced thin

1 red bell pepper, seeded and diced

1 green bell pepper, seeded and diced

1 small jalapeno pepper, seeded and minced

1 zucchini, seeded and diced

1 summer squash, seeded and diced

1 tablespoon ground cumin

1 tablespoon chili powder

2 teaspoons paprika

2 tablespoons almond meal

3 (15-ounce) jars Green Mountain Gringo Roasted Chile Salsa,* divided

2 cups tomato juice

3 tablespoons tomato paste

1 (15-ounce) can black beans, drained well

1 (15-ounce) can chickpeas, drained well, half kept whole, half roughly chopped

juice of 1 lemon

1 bunch fresh cilantro, roughly chopped

1 bunch greens onions, green and white parts, sliced thin

1 to 2 tablespoons salt

2 ripe avocados, for garnish, large diced

* Green Mountain Gringo salsas can be found in Whole Foods and other grocery stores.

1. Place a large soup pot over medium to high heat. Add the olive oil. Once heated, add the onion and cook for 3 to 5 minutes, stirring often, until the onions are soft and translucent.

2. Add the garlic along with the red and green bell peppers, and continue to cook over medium heat for another 3 to 5 minutes.

3. Add the jalapeno pepper, zucchini, and summer squash, and continue to cook until all of the vegetables have softened. Be

sure to season lightly with portions of 1 to 2 tablespoons of salt every time you add another vegetable to the pot during the cooking process.

4. Add the cumin, chili powder, and paprika to the vegetables and cook for 1 to 2 minutes.

5. Add the almond meal and cook for another 2 minutes. The almond meal will slightly thicken the chili, so be sure to stir often to prevent the vegetables from burning the bottom of the pot.

6. Next, puree 1 of the jars of Green Mountain Gringo Roasted Chili Salsa until it is smooth.

7. Add the pureed Green Mountain Salsa along with the 2 regular jars to the sautéed vegetables along with the tomato juice, tomato paste, black beans, the whole chickpeas, and the chopped chickpeas, and bring the chili to a simmer.

8. Once the chili comes to a simmer, place a lid on the pot and cook on low heat for about 45 minutes to allow all the flavors to come together. Be sure to stir often.

9. Add the lemon juice, cilantro, and green onions, and continue to cook on low heat for the last 5 minutes before serving.

10. Portion the chili into bowls and garnish with fresh diced avocado.

LEMONY SALMON WITH SWEET 'N' SPICY ROOTS

My friend Erinn showed up at my home recently with a bag full of ingredients from the farmer's market. The way Erinn coaxes flavors from food is nothing short of magical. If you don't eat fish, the root vegetables are still the bomb, packed with flavor and nutrients.
Here's what Erinn has to say: "I use everything fresh when possible. It just tastes better! If you're worried about the sugars, cut the sweet potatoes and substitute broccoli or another favorite. If you have no taste for the heat of the chilies, use less or remove seeds to tone it down." MAKES 2 TO 4 SERVINGS

For Veggies

3 tablespoons coconut oil

2 medium sweet potatoes, in ¾-inch cubes

1 medium turnip, in ½-inch cubes (about 1 cup)

2 golden beets

2 carrots, julienned

¾ teaspoon fresh peeled ginger, minced

2 cloves garlic, minced

1 medium red onion

½ teaspoon fresh turmeric, grated, or ¼ teaspoon ground tumeric

1 teaspoon apple cider vinegar

½ cup cabbage, coarsely shredded

½ cup kale (about 3 or 4 leaves), coarsely shredded

½ cup cremini mushrooms, sliced

2 Thai chilies, sliced lengthwise

½ teaspoon dried rosemary

1 teaspoon chopped Thai basil

cracked pepper and salt to taste

For Salmon

1 tablespoon butter, ghee, or coconut oil

2 green onions, sliced

¼ teaspoon grated fresh peeled ginger

juice of ½ lemon, divided

2 (5-ounce) salmon fillets

Veggies:

1. Heat the coconut oil in a large skillet or wok over medium heat until hot enough to bubble. Toss in a piece of beet to check.

2. Add the sweet potatoes, turnip, and beets all at once. Cook about 5 minutes, stirring frequently.

3. Add the carrots, ginger, garlic, onion, turmeric, and vinegar. Reduce the heat to just below medium. Cover and cook for 5 minutes.

4. Add the rest of the ingredients and simmer another 7 minutes.

Salmon:

If serving with the root vegetables, start this process during step 3 above.

1. Place the butter (or ghee, or coconut oil) in a medium pan and melt fully on medium heat.

2. Add the shallots, ginger and three-quarters of the lemon juice.

3. Simmer until translucent, then remove shallot-ginger mix from the pan and set aside, keeping the butter–lemon juice mixture in the pan.

4. Return the pan to medium heat and add the salmon, skin-side up to sear the fillets, about 5 minutes.

5. Flip the fillets over and pour the remaining lemon juice over the top. Cook 3 minutes.

6. Return the shallot and ginger to the pan. The salmon will become firm as it finishes cooking. Gently pull apart a few layers to make sure it's cooked through, and remove from the heat.

7. Serve the salmon with shallots and ginger over the top, with generous portions of veggies.

SERVING IDEAS

- Serve the vegetables warm over baby spinach for a hot salad.
- Use leftover veggies to make a spicy omelet.
- Heat up some veggie broth and stir in leftover vegetables for a quick pick-me-up soup.

SPICY COCONUT-CURRY LENTIL STEW

Erinn must have been a gourmet in his previous life. It's the only explanation for the amazing combination of flavors he pulls from food. That being said, I'm a simple cook and am always squabbling with Erinn over the 150 ingredients he insists on using. However, I lose the argument every time as there's no way around the fact that his food makes my mouth water. Since this recipe is labor-intensive, I'd suggest doubling it and freezing the extra in quart-size bags to pull out for a healthy on-the-go meal. MAKES 6 SERVINGS

2 pounds sweet potatoes (about 2 large sweet potatoes)

1 tablespoon olive oil

1 large onion, chopped

2 large carrots, chopped

1 medium turnip, in ¾-inch cubes (about ½ cup)

4 cloves garlic, chopped roughly

1 tablespoon grated fresh peeled ginger

1 tablespoon curry powder

½ tablespoon grated fresh turmeric

½ tablespoon salt

½ tablespoon freshly ground pepper

2 small green Thai chilies, sliced

2 cups vegetable broth

1½ cups green lentils

1 cup water

½ cup coconut cream

½ teaspoon ground cinnamon

4 big leaves of dinosaur kale (aka lacinato kale), chopped in ½-inch-wide ribbons

1 medium red bell pepper, sliced in ¼-inch-wide strips

sliced fresh tomato, for garnish

1. Peel one of the sweet potatoes and chop both potatoes into about 1-inch cubes. Set the peeled sweet potato aside.

2. Heat the olive oil in a large pot over medium heat. Add the onion, carrots, and the unpeeled sweet potato. Sauté until the onions begin to soften and become translucent, about 5 minutes.

3. Add the turnip, garlic, ginger, curry powder, turmeric, salt, and pepper, and sauté for 2 minutes longer, stirring constantly.

4. Add the Thai chilies, vegetable broth, and lentils, and bring to a boil over medium-high heat. Cover the pot, reduce the heat to medium-low, and simmer for 30 minutes, or until the lentils are tender.

5. While the lentils are simmering, boil the water in a medium pot over high heat. Stir in the peeled sweet potatoes and bring to a boil.

6. Reduce the heat to medium, cover, and cook until the sweet potatoes are very tender, about 10 minutes. (A fork should go in without effort.)

7. Drain the sweet potatoes, reserving 1 cup of the hot potato water aside for the puree. Place the sweet potatoes into a food processor. Add the coconut cream, reserved potato water, and cinnamon, and puree until smooth.

8. With 10 minutes left to simmer for the lentils, stir the kale and red bell pepper into the stew.

9. Test to make sure lentils are thoroughly cooked. Add the coconut-sweet potato puree to thicken—and add flavor!

10. Once the stew has thickened, just a few minutes, it's finished. Garnish with sliced, fresh tomatoes if desired and add salt to taste.

Note: Erinn is a runner and uses this recipe to replenish after a cold morning on the trail. In his own words, "You can play with this recipe for your taste. It doesn't have a lot of salt, but it does have a lot of flavor! I tend to leave veggies unpeeled and put the ones that cook fastest in just before the end because I like to keep them a bit crisp. You can omit the chili peppers or use less if you don't like it very hot. You can also use powdered ingredients and regular pepper, but the flavor is so much better to me when everything is fresh."

STUFFED EGGPLANT

For years, eggplant was my Everest. No matter what I did or how I treated it, my eggplant came out rubbery, slimy, or mushy. When I finally found a recipe that made eggplant taste good, I was over the moon. I now make the following recipe about once a week, eating it for breakfast, lunch, and dinner. SERVES 2

3 or 4 small eggplants or 1 large eggplant
3 tablespoons extra-virgin olive oil
½ red or yellow onion,* diced (2 to 4 cups)

assortment of chopped vegetables of your choosing: asparagus, broccoli, red/yellow/ orange bell peppers, mushrooms, etc.
4 cloves garlic, minced
1 to 2 tablespoons balsamic vinegar
salt and pepper

* I find using a red onion adds more flavor, but not everyone is a red onion fiend like me. If that's the case, a yellow onion works just fine.

Tip: Use a stainless steel knife to cut the eggplant. Carbon steel reacts with phytonutrients in the eggplant, causing it to turn black.

1. Preheat oven to 350°F.

2. Spray a baking sheet with coconut oil cooking spray and set aside.

3. Wash the eggplant(s) and cut off the ends. Slice in half lengthwise.

4. Use a small knife to remove the insides of the eggplant and chop. Set aside. Place the hollowed-out eggplant shells on the baking sheet.

5. In a large skillet or wok, heat the extra-virgin olive oil over medium heat.

6. Add the chopped vegetables, including the insides of the eggplant. Sauté until tender, 5 to 10 minutes.

7. Add the garlic and balsamic vinegar. Cook for another 1 to 2 minutes, until the garlic is fragrant. Season with salt and pepper to taste.

8. Spoon the vegetables into the eggplant shells.[27] Bake for 30 minutes.

SERVING IDEAS

- For a special treat, try stuffing the shells with chopped eggplant, roasted peppers, sun-dried tomatoes packed in olive oil, feta cheese, and pine nuts.

- Serve any extra vegetables over Basic Cauliflower Rice (page 148).

- Instead of using the hollowed-out eggplant shells, remove the gills from a portobello mushroom, brush the mushroom with extra-virgin olive oil, and stuff with the eggplant-veggie mixture. Bake as above, checking every 10 minutes for doneness.

---

27 I always find I have too many veggies to fit into the shells, which is an awesome problem to have. Simply save any extra sautéed veggies and add to your morning egg scramble for a delicious meal.

BAKED ONIONS

I love food you can stick in the oven and walk away from until it's time to pull it out and eat. However, I was not sold on the idea of eating an onion for a meal. That is, until I tasted a baked Vidalia onion. You can eat these plain or stuff them with goodies. Either way, it's a win. Also, your home will smell amazing while they're cooking! SERVES 1 TO 12 DEPENDING ON HOW MANY YOU MAKE!

1 Vidalia onion per person

2 cups stuffing of your choice—Cauliflower Rice (page 148) and veggies are a favorite of mine

1. Preheat the oven to 350°F.

2. Cut the tops off the onions and use a knife to core out each onion, leaving a thick wall to hold filling.

3. Fill the onions with a vegetable stuffing or a Paleo sauce of your choice (homemade Worcestershire, balsamic vinaigrette, etc.).

4. Wrap each onion individually in aluminum foil and place in a foil-lined baking dish.

5. Bake for 1 hour, until softened and slightly brown.

SERVING IDEAS

- Fill the onions with the Stuffed Eggplant mixture (page 164).

- Stuff with Basic Cauliflower Rice (page 148), black beans, and sun-dried tomatoes.

- If you're eating cheese, top with a small bit of goat cheese or feta when they come out of the oven.

- Save the cored-out onion center and chop or dice and use in other recipes.

Chapter 14

Fast & Easy Meals

Sometimes you just need to grab-n-go. These recipes are some of my favorite go-tos when I have limited time and/or interest in cooking.

EGG-AVOCADO SANDWICH

A ripe avocado can be used in place of mayonnaise in most recipes. Using it here makes for a great egg-salad recipe. SERVES 1

1 hard-boiled pasture-raised egg
½ very ripe avocado

1 red bell pepper, seeded and cut in half lengthwise
¼ cup baby spinach (optional)
salt and pepper

1. In a small bowl, use a fork to mash together the egg and avocado.
2. Season with salt and pepper to taste.
3. Stuff each pepper half with the egg-avocado mixture and top with the baby spinach.

SERVING IDEAS

- Serve the egg-avocado mixture on top of a salad.
- Spoon into celery for a snack.
- Makes a delicious sandwich on Paleo Bread (page 155)!

SWEET POTATO TOPPER

I enjoy even a plain sweet potato but the simple addition of nuts and butter makes it seem more like a meal. SERVES 1

1 sweet potato

1 teaspoon butter or ghee

handful of walnuts, chopped

1. Place the sweet potato on a microwave-safe plate and cook on high for about 7 minutes until tender.

2. Discard the potato skin and spread butter or ghee over the sweet potato.

3. Sprinkle with chopped walnuts.

SERVING IDEAS

- Add a handful of cooked or wilted baby spinach or other greens for added protein. Or, serve alongside a healthy portion of cooked greens.

- Top with ½ cup black beans and a few slices of avocado for a protein wallop.

SHREDDED CABBAGE CATCH-ALL

Probably the only recipe I use that relies on pre-packaged ingredients. You're welcome! SERVES 1

1 (6-ounce) bag shredded cabbage (I like the multicolored variety)

1 (4- to 6-ounce) can tuna or salmon, water-packed

1 tablespoon extra-virgin olive oil

lemon juice

salt and pepper

1. Combine all the ingredients in a bowl. Mix and serve.

SERVING IDEAS

- Include 6 pitted and halved kalamata olives.

- Toss in a small amount of slivered nuts.

- Include any chopped vegetables you have sitting around.

- Post-workout, add a few slices of green apple or a handful of grapes.

ZUCCHINI NOODLES

This is the PV answer to ramen noodles—fast, easy, and inexpensive. SERVES 1

1 large zucchini

1 teaspoon butter, ghee, or coconut oil

1. Use a vegetable peeler to peel the zucchini into long, thin strips.
2. Melt the butter, ghee, or coconut oil in a pan over medium-high heat.
3. Add the "noodles" and stir frequently for 2 to 5 minutes. The noodles should still be semi-firm.

SERVING IDEAS

- Treat as pasta and top with marinara sauce and veggies of your choice.
- Cook in olive oil and sprinkle with your favorite herbs, mushrooms, and sun-dried tomatoes.
- Top with veggies and a small bit of melted goat cheese.
- Toss with a Paleo-friendly pesto and add cherry tomatoes and fresh basil.

SLOW COOKER SQUASH

When my sister told me she cooked whole butternut squashes in her slow cooker, my reaction was "No. Way." Then I held her down and gave her a rug burn for lying. (Old sisterly habits die hard.) But it turns out my little sister knew what she was talking about. This is a ridiculously easy way to have squash on hand at any time. SERVES 2

   1 butternut squash

1. Place the whole squash in a slow cooker on low heat for 6 to 8 hours, or on high heat for 4 hours. No water required (seriously).

2. Remove the squash from the slow cooker. The squash will cut easily. Cube the squash and refrigerate until ready to serve.

SERVING IDEAS

- Serve with melted ghee or butter on top.
- Mash the cubed squash by hand or with a potato masher, add ghee, and serve as butternut squash mashed potatoes.
- Use in salads, stir-fries, and veggie sautés throughout the week.

PORTOBELLO MUSHROOM STEAKS

I can't live without portobellos. A big, juicy portobello mushroom is a meal in and of itself. Surround it with cauliflower mashed potatoes, a side of asparagus, and a hearty glass of red wine, and it's as fine a meal as you'll ever have. SERVES 2 TO 4

2 to 4 large portobello mushrooms

salt and pepper

1. Preheat the oven to 450°F.

2. Spray a baking sheet with coconut or olive oil cooking spray.

3. Clean the mushrooms with a damp paper towel.

4. Place the mushrooms on the baking sheet, gill-side up. Lightly season with salt and pepper to taste.

5. Roast for 15 to 25 minutes, checking occasionally, until the mushrooms are tender but not dried up.

SERVING IDEAS

- Top with marinara, baby spinach, and Italian seasoning.

- Top with crumbled blue cheese and baby spinach for last 5 minutes of roasting, allowing the cheese to melt.

- Top with your favorite chopped herbs and lemon juice or balsamic vinegar.

- Whisk together ⅓ cup balsamic vinegar, 1 tablespoon Dijon mustard, ¾ cup olive oil, and a little minced garlic. Baste the mushrooms with the mixture and place on a grill, gill-side up for 3 to 5 minutes. Flip, baste with a bit more of the liquid, and cook another 3 to 5 minutes until tender.

- Slice the cooked portobellos and layer into a red pepper for a "steak" sandwich.

Chapter 15

Sweet Treats

COCONUT CHOCOLATE BALLS

My friend Cindy is a beast. She is a competitive runner and tennis player, a fitness instructor, and runs an incredible gym. She is one of the healthiest eaters I know but that never stops her from indulging her sweet tooth. We invite Cindy to marathons not only for her upbeat personality but because we know she's going to show up with bags full of goodies for the ride there that are actually healthy. So it's no surprise when I was scouting around for PV recipes that Cindy sent me two for desserts. Enjoy these coconut chocolate balls adapted from OptimallyOrganic.com and the pumpkin streusel that follows. MAKES APPROXIMATELY 15 BALLS

1⅓ cups shredded coconut, divided

¼ cup coconut oil

2 tablespoons cacao powder (found in most health food stores)

1 tablespoon 100 percent pure maple syrup

chili powder

smoked paprika (optional)

1 teaspoon sea salt

1. Toast ⅓ cup of the shredded coconut. Spread on a microwave-safe plate and microwave on high for 2 to 3 minutes, stirring every 45 seconds. Or, bake at 325°F in the oven just until brown, about 10 minutes, checking constantly to be sure the coconut doesn't burn. Allow to cool.

2. Melt the coconut oil with the cacao powder over medium-low heat in a small saucepan.

3. Add ½ cup shredded coconut and the maple syrup. Stir until well mixed.

4. Add the chili powder and smoked paprika, if using, to taste. Again, stir until well mixed.

5. Remove from the pan and place in a medium bowl. Place in the freezer for at least 30 minutes but no more than 1 hour. You want the mixture to get firm but not completely frozen.

6. Meanwhile, mix the remaining ½ cup shredded coconut, the toasted coconut, and the salt together on a plate.

7. When the coconut-chocolate mixture is firm, remove the bowl from the freezer and use a tablespoon to scoop out the mixture and form them into loose balls with your hands.

8. Roll each ball in the shredded coconut and salt mixture, and enjoy.

PUMPKIN STREUSEL

If you're in this for weight loss, this recipe is more of a treat than a daily occurrence. But what's life without a taste of the sweet stuff? MAKES 12 SERVINGS

Crust

2 cups almond flour

3 tablespoons coconut oil, melted

1 teaspoon vanilla extract

1 tablespoon water

½ teaspoon salt

Filling

1 cup pumpkin puree

1 teaspoon ground cinnamon

½ teaspoon ground nutmeg

¼ teaspoon ground cloves

Streusel

3 tablespoons coconut oil, melted

1 tablespoon 100 percent pure maple syrup

¼ teaspoon salt

¼ teaspoon ground cinnamon

1 cup pecans, chopped

1. Preheat the oven to 350°F.

2. Spray an 8 x 8-inch baking dish with coconut oil cooking spray.

3. In a medium bowl, combine all the crust ingredients and stir well. Form the dough into a ball, then press it into an even layer in the bottom of the baking dish.

4. Bake for 10 minutes, until set, and then remove from the oven and allow to cool completely.

5. In a small bowl, stir together all the filling ingredients to combine. Spread the filling over the crust in a thin, even layer.

6. Mix together all the streusel ingredients except the pecans. Once combined, toss the pecans into the mixture and sprinkle over the top of the filling.

7. Bake everything together for 15 minutes, until set to the touch and pecans are just starting to brown. Be careful not to overcook and burn! Let cool for 10 minutes before serving.

Part III

Making the Paleo Vegetarian Lifestyle Work for You

Chapter 16

Balancing Your Diet, Sleep, and Exercise

Balancing Your Diet

I'm not a doctor and—sadly—I don't even get to play one on TV. For that reason, I'm gun-shy when it comes to giving advice on vitamins and supplements. I also believe there is no one-advice-fits-all standard for supplements. Some people are deficient in one area but strong in another. Paying attention to your body and how it feels and responds to what you ingest (often by trial and error) is the only real way to "know" what's right for you. For that reason, I'm going to offer you broad strokes when it comes to supplements and let you fill in the blanks.

Good health is all about self-monitoring. If I'm tired or run down or have no energy, I start paying close attention to my diet and sleep patterns. Am I not getting enough iron, or do I simply need more sleep? Am I spending at least a little time in the sun each day to boost my vitamin D, or is all my time spent indoors?

Our eating doesn't exist in a vacuum outside of everything else in our world. You can eat to perfection every day but still feel run down because you're not doing things like getting enough sleep, spending time outdoors, or making time to move and have fun. It's all tied in together.

It's funny—I was about to write, "Do you want to be thin if it means you're going to be miserable?" when I had a reality check. For way too many years I was chunky and I know during that time period I would have answered that question with a resounding, "Yes. Yes, I want to be thin even if it means I'm miserable because I believe being thin will bring me the happiness I want in life."

I'm older (and thinner) now, and I can say that while being healthy, fit, and thin does absolutely add to my pleasure in life, it is by no means a fix-all. There will always be job stress, relationship issues, the cat puking again on the front hall carpet...

In other words, life will always be there. So while it's fine to strive for fit and healthy, don't get so bogged down in the quest for perfection that you miss all the great things in life going on around you. Look at the people around you that matter. Would you feel different about them—better—if they dropped 5.5 pounds? No? Well, guess what. They probably won't love you any more or less if you're not at your goal weight. Just something to keep in mind.

So getting back to the point at hand, where do sleep and supplements come in? As a vegetarian, you're most susceptible to iron, calcium, and protein deficiencies. "Talk to your doctor before starting this or any diet/exercise program" sounds like a cop-out, but it's not a bad idea. They know you, know your body, and if you make it clear this is how you're choosing to eat, they can help point out where there might be nutritional deficiencies. Meanwhile, below are a few broad guidelines to get you started.

PROTEIN

The way I track my protein is through my weight, using Mark Sisson's method from MarksDailyApple.com. In Mark's words:

> At a minimum you need 0.5 grams of protein per pound of lean mass per day on average to maintain your "structure." If you are moderately active you need 0.7 or 0.8, and if you are an active athlete you need as much as 1 gram of protein per pound of lean mass. That's at a minimum, but it's on a daily average. So a 155-pound moderately active woman who has 25 percent body fat [28] and thus has 116 pounds of lean body mass needs 93 grams of protein [29] on average per day (116 x .8).

You may be saying to yourself, that seems like a crazy amount of protein. And it is, compared to standard dietary guidelines. But let's face it: The food pyramid has always been a step behind the times. This is a high-fat, high-protein, low- to medium-carb diet. And yes, it can be a challenge to hit that protein number, especially without meat as an easy and available protein source. That's why it's so important to track your protein intake, at least initially, to make sure you're coming close to getting what you need. Otherwise, you'll be left feeling hungry and tired.

CARBOHYDRATES

Again, we turn to Mark Sisson. Mark suggests 100 to 150 grams of carbohydrates per day for people who are at their preferred weight and body composition. If you're trying to lose weight, keep your carbs to less than 100 grams/day. If you are a heavy exerciser (loosely defined as training hard for more than one hour a day),

---

28 Calculate BMI by dividing weight in pounds (lbs) by height in inches (in) squared and multiplying by a conversion factor of 703.

29 That's the equivalent of about 14 large eggs. http://www. marksdailyapple.com/definitive-guide-to-the-primal-eating-plan/#ixzz3lZfH2vMp

you'll need to throw more carbs onto the mix. Mark suggests a guideline of up to 100 grams extra carbs/day for every additional hour you train over one hour.

SUGAR

To be honest, the only thing I am careful to always track in my diet is my sugar intake. If I control my sugar, I control my carbs. If I'm controlling my carbs, that means I'm eating plenty of other healthy fat- and protein-based foods to fill me up. For me, everything comes down to sugar, and I find it much, much easier to track just this one thing versus trying to create a macro flowchart of my dietary intake every single day.[30]

What follows is probably the greatest single weight-loss tip I can offer to anyone, PV, pure Paleo, vegetarian, or other. Here it is: *If you want to lose weight, keep your sugar intake under 20 grams per day.*

If you want to lose weight, keep your sugar intake under 20 grams per day.

That's it. Stay true to this one rule of thumb and it's almost impossible for the pounds *not* to come sliding off. That's not to say it doesn't require discipline. Consider, for example, that an apple or banana has close to that amount of sugar in a single serving. Even an egg has 1 gram of sugar. But high fat and high protein and lots of veggies translates to very little sugar, meaning you can eat to satiation and still lose the weight.

---

30 I would recommend when you start out that you track your protein intake as well. Once you've got a handle on that, you can focus more exclusively on sugar as suggested here.

IRON

Nuts and seeds contain iron, although not enough for you to get your daily intake, approximately 50 mg per day.[31] Infuse your diet with other iron-rich plant foods like Swiss chard and collard greens, mushrooms, and tomato sauce (watch for added sugars). Also, have you ever read that cooking with a cast-iron skillet boosts your iron intake? Turns out it's true. Plus, have you ever *lifted* a cast-iron skillet? I'm pretty sure cooking with one of those hefty bad boys counts as an upper-body workout.

CALCIUM

Contrary to what the rest of America believes, you don't have to partake in dairy to hit your daily calcium requirement. Tons of vegetables are rich in calcium, and as these will form the basis of many of your meals, you should be in good shape. Some of my favorites include collards, kale, sweet potatoes, butternut squash, turnip greens, almond butter, broccoli and fennel.[32]

VITAMIN D

Vitamin D deficiency is widespread in America. A simple way to counteract this is to get more sun. Mark Sisson recommends 20 minutes of sunlight each day without (brace yourselves) sunscreen. If that's not possible, a vitamin D supplement is a good idea. But make an effort to get outside, breathe some fresh air, and stand or go for a walk in the sun.

---

31 At least, not without ballooning up in weight due to the amount you'd need to eat.

32 If you've never roasted raw fennel in your oven you are missing out on a heavenly aroma filling your home. Drizzled with just a bit of olive oil— delicious!

Sleep

Get your zzz's. This point is non-negotiable. Lack of sleep causes stress in the body and leads to an "alarmist" state where your body hangs on to every calorie and bit of fat as a defense mechanism. You might be able to battle your way through and get *really* strict with your diet to even out the lack of sleep, but you're still doing more harm than good. Everyone needs a good seven to eight hours of sleep a night, period. Getting enough sleep makes you more alert, improves your workouts, and makes you less hungry throughout the day. That's right, sleep deprivation is strongly linked to feelings of being constantly hungry and overeating throughout the day.

Rearranging our schedules to ensure we're getting the proper amount of sleep can be as life-altering as changing our diet. Speaking from personal experience, this is an area where I really struggled. I'm usually at the gym by 5:15 or 5:30 every morning, which means I'm up around 4:30. This gives me a bedtime of about 9 p.m. when there are things I feel I need to be doing, like laundry and e-mails and spending time with the cat.

Like everything in life, choosing to get enough sleep is just that: a choice. There are still some days where I only get five to six hours and I feel every minute of it during the day. And yes, on those days it seems like I can't get enough food in my system. So I chose to go to bed early or—and this was a hard one for me—I've learned to recognize that I'll be better off in the long run choosing an extra two hours of sleep over doing a sleep-deprived cardio workout that burns 800 calories. For most of my life, I've been programmed to suck it up and do the workout because calorie burn is where it's at. Folks, we've been lied to. Exercise is not the magic elixir to losing weight.

Let's take a closer look at why that is.

Exercise

Don't act so surprised. You knew this was coming. Has there ever been a diet book in the history of the earth that didn't include the obligatory section on exercise? My favorites are a couple of straight-up Paleo cookbooks I own with nothing but recipes—and 20 pages in the back on the proper technique to do standing lunges, chair dips, and flys. Stir the sauce, but drop and give me ten push-ups before you add the pepper. Classic!

Here's the good news. I'm not here to teach you technique or to guilt you into exercising. When it comes to losing weight—and remember when we say we want to lose weight what we really mean is we want to lose *fat*—diet alone will get you 80 percent of the way there. Can I get an "Amen!" from the crowd?

The mainstream media is just now catching on to this. For decades we've been told that cardio three times a week is the key to losing weight. Instead, it turns out all that cardio did little more than to make us hungry. Especially as we were filling up before and after our workouts on "protein" or "granola" bars that were (and still are) the nutritional equivalent of eating a Snickers.

The purpose of this book is to advise you on how to start and maintain a Paleo Vegetarian diet. Whether you chose to incorporate exercise into that plan is up to you. The beauty of a PV diet is that you can maintain or lose weight without exercise. This isn't to say that exercise isn't beneficial. You're not going to get a super-toned, lean, muscle-y body just sitting on the couch.[33] But that may not be your goal. You may just want to feel good in your clothes and in your life. Or you may feel the need to only tackle one major challenge at a time, and changing up your diet comes first. After you're good with that, you'll move your attention to exercise.

---

33 Damn it.

I know, however, there are a lot of you out there who are already dedicated or even hardcore exercisers. We need to have a little discussion around that. You may be astounded, surprised, or shocked (or even ticked off) when I tell you that you may be going at this exercise/weight loss thing the wrong way. In fact, especially if you're what the Paleo world refers to as a "chronic cardio" person, your workouts may actually be what's holding you back from losing weight instead of moving you toward your goal.

How can this be? Let's think about the different types of exercise. There's everything from "couch-potato mode" where you do no movement, to performing average, everyday "life" movements like walking to your car or carrying in groceries, to moderate exercise such as hitting the gym a couple of times a week or power walking, to those people you see on the TV exercise infomercials with crazed, bulging eyes to match their crazed, bulging muscles. We'll call them "hardcore."

Levels of Exercise

None/couch potato

Basic living

Moderate—power walking, gym class, easy bike ride or hike

Intense—One-hour power workouts, weight training, interval training

Hardcore—Over one hour per day of exercise, including intense cardio multiple times a week

Where do you fit on the spectrum? I hope you realize by now that feeling guilty—"I'm only basic but I should be intense!"—is not only a waste of time, but the negativity can cause adverse effects on your body. Stress, even self-induced, pumps cortisol into your system that triggers your body into a defensive mode. There should not be stress here, especially when you now know that you don't *have* to exercise to lose weight. Yes, exercise goes far beyond weight loss in terms of improving heart health and circulation, and releasing endorphins, which make us feel good. Exercise is important. But it's not the focus of this book.

Coming clean, I fall into the highly intense to hardcore categories, depending on if I'm training for a marathon or ultra event. I recognize, however, that I work out too much. Exercising as much as I do to train for ultras and marathons puts me at risk. My body is constantly under stress. Luckily, I recognize this and am able to take actions to compensate.

Whether you're a fitness demon or beginner exerciser, there are really only three things you must do in order to get the best performance and life out of your body. Here they are, in order of importance:

- Eat right
- Get plenty of sleep
- Lift heavy things occasionally

Ta-dah! Doesn't sound that hard, does it? And it isn't. We like to overcomplicate or overthink things and, sometimes, analysis can be fun. (You're talking to the girl who has tracked the mileage on each pair of running shoes she owns for the past nine years.) But when you have those moments where you're feeling overwhelmed, dial it back to basics. Eat right. Get your sleep. These two things alone will catapult (yes, *catapult*) you into good health. Adding in some occasional strength training is the sugar-free icing on the gluten-free cake that will shape your body and bring on additional health.

I can't emphasize the importance of these three items enough. I mentioned above that chronic cardio of the type I do places a constant stress on the body. My way of compensating for all that stress is to—you guessed it—eat right, get plenty of sleep, and do strength training to balance out the muscle groups being worked in my body.

But what does eating right for an athlete look like? And what constitutes being "an athlete" to begin with? Let's take a look.

AM I AN ATHLETE?

Let me tell you a story. This past summer, my friend Christie and I signed up to pace the two-hour group for a local half-marathon. When it comes to being loving and touchy-feely, Christie is a 30 on a 10-point scale. She lives to nurture. Me, not so much. The joke among our friends was that Christie would offer the "You all are doing wonderful, I'm so proud of each of you!" pep talks to the runners in our pace group while I would be behind the group screaming, "Why are you crying?! Run faster, b**ches!"[34]

I tell that story to share that I am in no way a touchy-feely person. And yet I hold the unshakable belief that anyone who shows up for the workout is an athlete. Whether you're winning races or simply walking on the treadmill at the gym once or twice a week, you've got your game on. Anyone who exercises understands that working out is not the hard part. It's *showing up* for the workout

---

34 True story: My office requires everyone take a personality test before hiring. The CEO sat down with me to go over my results and he was whipping through them, "Self-motivated. Good. Strong attention to detail. Good," when he came to an abrupt stop. He looked at me, looked at the page, looked back at me. "So," he said. "Nurturing. Uh, you scored a 7 out of 100." To this day, friends and coworkers refer to me as "Seven."

that requires fortitude. I've been running for almost ten years and yes, there are many, many days where I have to drag, beg, plead, and cajole myself to show up. I'm always glad I did, as I inevitably feel great once I've got a few miles under my feet, but the struggle never entirely goes away.

So before I dive into PV eating for athletes, I want to be clear that, as a former couch potato, I have complete and utter respect for anyone who is doing any level of exercise. With that said, as we talk about how to modify the PV diet for athletes, I am referring to a specific level of exercise. Namely, you'll need to make modifications and allowances in your diet if you're someone who *exercises at a high-intensity level for over an hour at a time or if you're completing intense or hardcore workouts several days a week.* If you're someone who performs low to moderate workouts, you shouldn't need to vary your eating other than allowing for a few more carbs on heavy workout days.

PRE-WORKOUT TIPS

Even for high-intensity workouts, you'd be surprised how little food you need to complete a workout. As a runner, I had it drummed into me that I needed to carbo-load the night before a run and eat a solid carbohydrate-based meal a couple of hours before the run as well. It took a long time for me to drop that mindset. And really the only thing that changed my mind was experimenting and seeing firsthand how my runs and workouts didn't suffer, and even improved, all without the carbo load.

Now, I eat a normal meal the night before a long (even 20 miles) run. I'm careful to make sure my meal contains protein and maybe some extra fat (More avocado? Yes, please), but I don't eat huge portions and I certainly don't load up on pasta and bread.

What really opened my eyes was working out in the fasted state. I always, always, always made sure to eat before any type of workout, strength or cardio. I thought I'd lose energy midworkout without the boost from food. But once I began intermittent fasting (see page 199), I ended up doing a couple of CrossFit workouts in the fasted state and—to my great surprise—I crushed them.

This isn't to say you need to fast before a workout. But it does give you some freedom in that you know you don't have to calorie load before a workout. If you prefer to eat before exercising, try to give yourself at least one to two hours in between a snack and your workout. A good pre-workout should be low on the glycemic index, so avoid fruit. A hard-boiled egg, a small cup of soup, or a small salad are all good choices.

Here are some tips I've tried that have worked well for me.

- A small cup of soup or broth an hour before a workout is satisfying and can stave off hunger during the workout.

- Eliminate carbo-loading. If you're an endurance athlete, you might up your fat and carb uptake gradually in the week before your race, but training with your regular PV diet should be enough to get you through your workout.

- Don't use exercise as an excuse to reward yourself with food. This often happens with cardio workouts. The machine tells us we just burned 500 calories so we splurge and go eat a 480-calorie bagel or a smoothie with 30 grams of sugar. No, no, and no.

- A tablespoon of almond butter before a workout sticks to the stomach without weighing you down.

- I'm a huge fan of sweet potatoes as a healthy source for carbs. I'll eat a small sweet potato before a long run or follow up my run with a sweet potato covered in butter or ghee.

- Try exercising in the fasted state and note the results. Did you have more or less energy?

- If you're exercising at a high-intensity level for more than an hour, you'll need to replenish midworkout. Please don't rely on GUs and energy drinks that are filled with sugar and fake ingredients. Instead, bring a piece of fruit and some almond butter. I (no surprise) still like my sweet potato. I'll microwave one in the morning and scoop the insides into a little baggie that I'll carry with me on a long run. A hard-boiled egg is an easy-to-carry-along snack as well.

POST-WORKOUT TIPS

For endurance workouts that last over an hour, you'll want to replenish with foods that have a 5:1 carb-to-protein ratio. For hard workouts, post-workout is the time when you can fudge a bit on the PV diet and go heavier on the carbs and sugar, as your body is in high-burn mode.

If you've done hard cardio, it's okay to replenish the body with something like a banana or apple smeared with almond butter, or a hard-boiled egg and some dried (no-sugar-added) fruit. Sweet potato pancakes or any starchy vegetable such as squash, turnips, pumpkin, or yams are great post-workout choices. If you eat fish, a little smoked salmon is an ideal protein source, even better if it's eaten alongside a carb source.

After a workout you want to focus more on carbs and protein. Save the fat for later meals. Why? You're trying to get the carbs and protein absorbed into your system as quickly as possible, and fats slow down that process. Try to eat within 30 minutes of completing your workout, as the body is most susceptible to absorbing nutrients during that window. That's when the post-fuel food aids in replenishing tired and depleted muscles.

Bear in mind that your need for replenishment will vary by individual and workout type. A one-hour yoga workout or 20 minutes of light weights won't require anywhere near the same replenishment as 45 minutes on the bike or a super-heavy 30-minute weight-lifting session. Again, experiment, experiment, experiment to find out what works best for you.

Simple grab-on-the-go foods for the 30-minute post-workout recovery window include:

- Banana or apple with almond butter
- Handful of raisins or berries
- Small sweet potato with a hard-boiled egg on the side
- Mashed sweet potato mixed with pure, unsweetened, organic applesauce
- Fried or scrambled eggs alongside Paleo toast with ghee, butter, or avocado spread
- Any roasted root vegetables (turnips, parsnips, butternut squash, etc.) with a side of sautéed greens
- PV Pancakes (page 147)
- Cup of Spicy Coconut-Curry Lentil Stew (page 162)

IF YOU REALLY WANT A NUMBER...

I know, I know. If you're like me, you don't want to be told to experiment. You want guidelines. Okay. On average, when I'm trying to lean out and shed some weight, I aim to keep my sugars under 20 grams per day and my carbs under 120 grams. However, on the days I do heavy cardio, I'll allow up to 100 extra grams of carbs. On heavy weight-lifting days, I'll allow up to an extra 50. I've found I can do this and maintain my weight or even lose weight (fat). On heavy exercise days I still try to keep my sugars around 20 grams, but this number does go up slightly if I'm eating more sweet potato or fruit due to a big workout.

If you're determined (like me) to indulge in the chronic cardio, it's important you add those extra carbs so you don't stress your body out. Deprive it of the replenishment it needs and it will react by holding on to fat. If you're starting out at a much lower or beginning level of exercise, hold off on adding extra carbs to your diet. Once you transform from sugar-burning to fat-burning, you ought to have plenty of energy and resources available to you on that 120 to 150 grams of carbs per day base level.

Please use the above only as a guideline. You're a different weight, height, body build, and probably exercise intensity level from me. What works for me may not be ideal for you. But start here and play with carb ratios until you find your sweet spot where you have plenty of energy to get through your workouts, feel satiated by your post-workout meals, and are still losing weight.

ONE MORE WORD ON EXERCISE AND EATING

Before we leave the world of eating and exercise, I must emphasize this fact: Have a plan. I can't tell you the number of times I've made poor food choices after a workout simply because I failed to plan ahead. Running 18 miles and then walking into a bagel shop? Recipe for disaster. Now I know to make sure I have the right kinds of foods available to me after my workouts. I keep a bunch of hard-boiled eggs in the fridge. The day before an intense workout, I'll go to the store and buy an apple to carry in my gym bag alongside some almond butter. I'll even cook an omelette or roast a sweet potato and asparagus the night before a workout so I can come home, heat the food up in my microwave, and have a delicious and filling post-workout meal at hand. Premade vegetable frittatas are also really fun and a delicious option for a post-recovery meal. And here's a down-and-dirty trick for when you're really pressed for time—canned pumpkin. That's right, you heard it here first.

If you're starting to feel overwhelmed, take a deep breath and go back to the three basics: Eat right, get plenty of sleep, and lift some weights a couple of times a week. Keep it that simple.

What I've learned from this journey is that our bodies are amazingly adaptable. When fueled on an ongoing basis with high-quality whole foods, we don't need all the extra sugars and food fillers to "get us through" a workout. Instead, our bodies remain in a highly prepared and energy-laden state.

To our health!

Chapter 17

When the Scale Won't Budge: Diet Tips, Hacks, and Modifications

Your body is an ongoing experiment. Furthermore, no two bodies are exactly alike. Why do you and your bestie follow the same eating plan and she loses weight and you don't? Is it because she sucks? Maybe. But a more reasonable response to the weight loss mystery is that the two of you have different bodies with different needs that will respond in different ways.

To that end, we all may find ourselves "stuck" at different points along the journey, sometimes due to factors beyond our control and sometimes because we backslid in our intentions. Both are normal and to be expected. After all, do you know *anyone* who consistently loses weight week after week after week with no plateau or backlash? (Hint: If you do, you need to stop being friends with that person. Instantly.) Our bodies, minds, and emotions take time to adjust to a new mode of eating. What can help is having tools in our healthy-eating arsenal so that when those backslides or sticking points occur, a fix is within easy reach.

You can use the tips and modifications below on an as-needed basis or incorporate them as regular aspects into your diet. Just remember, slow and steady. Take it from a type A perfectionist, attempting to do everything all at once, perfect from the get-go, is almost always a path that leads straight to Ben & Jerry's binge eating when the plans go awry. Instead, ease up, cut yourself some slack, and feel your way through those rough patches.

PAY ATTENTION TO THE FOOD THAT YOU EAT. Well, duh. Isn't that what we've been talking about this whole time? Sort of. Except now I'm talking less about the selection of foods and more about the actual experience of eating. It's a pain in the you-know-what, but being mindful of every bite that goes in your mouth is a truly excellent weight-loss tool that will fill you up faster and keep you satiated longer. I can eat the exact same breakfast of a veggie-scramble mix in the morning, and if I sit at the table and focus on my food, I'm full for hours. If I shovel the meal in while I read an article from *The New Yorker,* it's almost as if I'd never eaten. Which typically leads to my eating more or starting off the day grumpy because I just ate a big breakfast and it wasn't enough. So yes, put down the iPad and turn off the TV. You'll feel fuller and eat less in the long run if you sit down and focus exclusively on eating.

DRINK MORE WATER. I can feel you rolling your eyes. Oh sheesh, this again? Yup, this again, only with a slight twist. I don't think the standard "Drink eight 8-ounce glasses of water a day" adage holds true. We may not need that much water. But you probably do need more than you're getting. Often what we mistake for hunger is actually our body telling us it's dehydrated. When you have the urge to snack, drink a glass of water and wait ten minutes. If you're still hungry, go ahead and eat. But you may find that water was what your body was craving and you don't actually need to eat.

MIX UP YOUR MEALS. What do I mean when I say mix up your meals? Essentially I'm asking you to break the mindset of what is normal and "acceptable" for breakfast, lunch, and dinner. Why is this important? It's going to give you a lot more freedom and flexibility in what you prepare, which hearkens back to those feelings of abundance we discussed earlier.

We've all known the joys of eating breakfast for dinner. Is there anything better than a stack of hot pancakes with real butter (or ghee) running down the sides at 7 o'clock at night? (There are Paleo pancakes. Check out the super-simple mashed-banana Paleo pancake recipe on page 147.) I love pancakes, but my morning routine doesn't leave time for them. I'm lucky if I have time to peel and wolf down a hard-boiled egg. So I make them for dinner instead.

If I'm eating pancakes for dinner, I may as well eat my dinner food at 6 a.m. And so I do. On a regular basis, I sit down to a morning meal that consists of something along the lines of roasted cauliflower steak, asparagus, and sautéed spinach with shaved pecans. Dinner leftovers are delicious in the a.m., full of unexpected spices and flavor, and the best part is, you don't have to cook! Pop last night's dinner into the microwave for 45 seconds and enjoy it as a delicious hot breakfast.

KEEP MEALS SIMPLE. Don't you just love diet books that offer up seven to ten different menu options for every meal? Where exactly are people working that they have the time (and access to a stove) to prepare homemade enchiladas during their lunch hour? And who has time to mix anything in a bowl let alone bake something in the morning? I mean, seriously? Tim Ferriss said it best: "Eat the same meal over and over." Embrace the beauty of the "go-to" meal, one you know how to prepare quickly and that you know you like. Eat the same simple meal often and save the stress of innovative cooking for the days when you have the time and inclination.

BE MINDFUL OF HOW YOU THINK ABOUT FOOD. Food should not be a reward (I earned this peanut-butter granola bar!) or a punishment (I've been so bad on my diet that I'm not eating anything for the next 24 hours). Unfortunately, most of us have spent our lives thinking of food exactly as that. The undoing of years of "bad thought" food training takes time, but it's worth the effort. When you finally start looking at food as nourishment instead of slotting it into "can have/can't have" categories, it's world-changing. So much so that you may find that changing the way you think about food also changes the way you think about life. You'll become more conscious of all the choices in life that are available to you. Don't be surprised when this new and healthy way of thinking about food spills over into your cheat days. The first couple times you "earn" a cheat day, it will be like *Girls Gone Wild,* only with food. After the benefits of feeling good all week on the PV diet kick in, however, you'll stop thinking of cheat days as something you've "earned," and voluntarily dial them back to perhaps enjoying a good meal or eating more fruit than usual. You may even find there are weeks where you feel no need for the cheat day.

PAY ATTENTION TO HOW YOU TALK ABOUT FOOD. For me, this involved losing the mindset that food is bad or something that must be rationed. It took my 70-year-old mother talking to me on the phone one day as she was trying to lose weight and hearing her say, "Now, apples are bad for me, right?" to snap me to attention. Now I listen to my words when I talk about food to make sure they reflect my true intentions.

MAKE THE DIET FIT YOUR LIFESTYLE VERSUS CHANGING YOUR LIFESTYLE TO FIT THE DIET. Your food preparation and eating choices shouldn't be filling your mind every second of the day. If they are, that means something about your diet isn't working for you. Yes, there will be times when you're prepping food for meals that will feel all-encompassing and you'll need to monitor your protein and sugar intake, but what you can, should, and will eat should not be the focal point of your days. There's more to life than eating a perfect diet.

BEWARE OF EATING "HEALTHY" CRAP. Fess up—most of us began our foray into vegetarianism with some form of the "ice cream and cereal for dinner" mindset. If it wasn't meat, it was "safe" and counted as part of a vegetarian diet. Teenage vegetarians who exist on Doritos and Taco Bell bean burritos exemplify this. But we wised up, found some simple recipes, learned how to pronounce "quinoa," discovered Amy's and MorningStar foods, and transitioned into a healthier mode of meat-free eating.

There are a number of foods out there that claim to be Paleo. And, just as Doritos are technically vegetarian, these other foods are technically Paleo. However, check out the sugar grams on some of those "Paleo-friendly" products. I looked at a Paleo brownie the other day that had 17.9 grams of sugar. A Betty Crocker brownie has 17.1! You can eat these Paleo products and not technically be "cheating," but you're not going to lose weight doing it.

MAKE SURE YOU'RE EATING ENOUGH. Go ahead, say it. Best diet tip, ever. How do you make sure you're getting enough to eat? Tracking your energy levels is a good starting point. You should not feel hungry, deprived, tired, drained, or miserable. You should feel light, energized, awake, and alert. If you're not feeling this way, take a couple of days and track your calories—not in the interest of limiting them, but in the interest of making sure you're eating enough. And not just enough food in general, but enough of the right types of foods. Eat plenty of fats, as these will boost your energy levels. Especially track your protein as the vegetarian part of the PV equation takes away a significant Paleo source of protein—meat. It may also help to note how eating different types of food makes you feel. For example, eating an apple before a workout made me feel full, but I find I have a better workout if I eat fat (nut butter or an avocado) instead of fructose and carbs.

GIVE INTERMITTENT FASTING (IF) A TRY. I've never been a fan of fasting. I don't like skipping meals. Not so much because I'm hungry, but because it goes back to that feeling of deprivation. That, and I'm the poster child for reverse psychology. Tell me I can eat anything and I'll shrug and say I'm not hungry or I can wait. Tell me I have to fast and it's guaranteed I'll be salivating outside the fridge 20 minutes after polishing off a large meal.

That being said, I've taken to the concept of intermittent fasting. I find it one of the fastest and—truly—easiest ways to jump-start weight loss. The theory behind IF, as it's known, is that it's easier to fast for one day to reduce your weekly caloric intake rather than discipline yourself to cut back on 500 calories every day.

There are a couple of tricks to engaging in successful IF. Rule number one—no gorging! There's no need (and you're missing the point) if you load up on food both before and after a fast. IF is about eating your normal daily intake, pausing for a set amount of time, then eating normally again.

Once your body has switched over to fat-burning versus sugar-burning, you'll be able to handle 12 hours of fasting, no problem. This is especially true if you plan your fast so you're asleep for most of it. If you eat a late lunch, your fast may only involve skipping dinner and then eating a late breakfast.

Ease into IF. Many Paleo websites talk about doing a 24-hour intermittent fast one to two times per week. I find a once-a-week fast of 16 to 18 hours serves just fine to keep my weight in check. Experiment and find what works for you, but remember the key word here is "intermittent." You shouldn't be fasting every other day. PV is not about extended caloric restriction. IF is a simple tool to jump-start weight loss. It's not even a must-do.

A SAMPLE IF PLAN

What I've found that works for me is eating a late lunch, around 3 or 4 p.m., and then starting the fast. I make sure my lunch contains plenty of healthy fats and protein to keep hunger at bay but, again, I don't overeat. A protein-laden meal is more than capable of keeping me full until at least 8 p.m. and then it's just a matter of making it an hour or two until bedtime. By the time I wake up at 5 a.m., I'm already 13 hours into the fast. And—being a fat-burning machine—I find I'm rarely hungry, even during an IF, when I wake up in the mornings.

If you feel hungry, drink plenty of water, coffee, tea. Soda isn't Paleo due to all the added sugars, and even diet soda is off limits as it has no nutritional value and contains non-whole-food ingredients. If you're not a fan of plain water, sparkling water (also called soda water) is Paleo-friendly. Avoid the flavored versions but feel free to add mint, cucumber, or lemons for a burst of fresh flavor.

Stay busy. Run errands, clean the house, do some work—anything you don't associate with eating. Try to go for 16 hours. If you need to, munch on four or five almonds, and eat each one slowly and thoughtfully. You'll be surprised, after having not eaten for 12 hours, how filling a couple of almonds can be. Then break the fast with a late breakfast at around 10 a.m. Boom! Your first 16-hour fast, over and done with. And, really, the only meal you skipped was dinner.

If you're so inclined, extend the fast up to 24 hours. I usually play around with the 16-to-20-hour fast, and that works for me. You'll need to experiment and see what works for you. Also, remember that breaking the fast isn't cause to eat everything in sight. Eat what you normally would for breakfast or lunch, drink plenty of water and continue on with the PV diet, eating when you're hungry (instead of eating by the clock) for your next meal.

CONDENSE YOUR EATING INTO AN EIGHT-HOUR PERIOD.
This is actually another version of intermittent fasting. The idea is to eat only within an 8-hour window each day, which more or less forces you into a 16-hour fast for the remaining time period.

I personally find this difficult to do given my work schedule, but it works for some people (including Hugh Jackman, who used IF and restrictive eating to lose weight and bulk up for his *Wolverine* roles).

COOK ONCE AND THEN COOK A LOT. We're back to bulk cooking. I suspect I'm preaching to the choir on this one, but just in case you're unfamiliar with the joys of bulk cooking, allow me to enlighten you one more time. It pretty much comes down to basic math: 1 mess + 1 time = 8 meals. Of course, if you have the time and inclination to prepare food daily or set time aside to cook healthy for each and every meal, Godspeed. But most of us are overburdened with the demands on our time, including work, house, spouse, kids, pets, parents, PTA, workouts, volunteer activities, and catching up on *Game of Thrones* and *House of Cards* to bother with cooking every night.

The point is, when you finally do find the time to cook, go ahead and COOK. Double or triple the side item or main dish you're preparing so you'll have plenty of meal options for the next few days and won't be tempted to pay $2 for the canola oil–laden peanut butter granola bar in the vending machine at work.

EXERCISE MORE. Or less. I've been accused of being a compulsive exerciser. I like to work out, and when I do, I like to go after it hard. I've got it under control now, but for way too many years, I had a fear of not working out. Skipping even one workout meant weight gain in my mind. It got to a point where I was working out five or six days a week, usually twice a day, with CrossFit in the morning and tempo or long runs in the afternoon. I was eating all the right foods but found myself frustrated as I watched the scale inch its way in the wrong direction.

It was only when I cut back on exercise—especially cardio—that the weight came off. I suspect all the exercise—and the lack of sleep from getting up for 5 a.m. CrossFit workouts—was negatively affecting my cortisol levels. The resulting stress and inflammation threw my body into "survivor" mode where it clung to fat, literally because it sensed it was being attacked.

If you're not doing any or only minimal exercise and your weight loss has stalled, it's probably time to take it up a notch. Bodyweight exercises and lifting heavy things (in lieu of cardio) is extremely effective for revving up your metabolism and keeping the fires burning, even when you're at rest.

However, if you're a hardcore exerciser, and especially if you do a lot of cardio, play around with doing less. Take it down to three days a week instead of five or six, and, again, focus more on weight training instead of cardio. Like me, you may be surprised at the results.

GO TO BED. We've already discussed the importance of sleep in being healthy and regulating your body's functions. There are new studies every day showing that lack of sleep plays a major role in people not being able to lose weight. We're a country that prides ourselves on our ability to get by on four to five hours a night, but at what cost to our health? Lack of sleep stresses the body, causing inflammation and, just like too much exercise, makes your body think it must go into defense mode and hang on to fat. More sleep equals less stress equals a responsive body. Sleep isn't an option when it comes to good health and losing weight—it's a necessity. Make it happen.

REMIND YOURSELF WHY YOU'RE DOING THIS. What's your reason for trying the PV diet? Is it because you want to be healthy or you're aiming for a Victoria Secret–like body—or both? There's nothing wrong with wanting to be thin and toned. It's almost impossible not to want it giving the daily deluge of "you must be thin with perfect hair, nails, home, and children" messages we are assaulted with on a daily basis. And I'd be lying if I said I hadn't tried diets over the years not to be healthy, but solely because I wanted to shed the pounds.

I hope, however, you're willing to factor in your health to any diet you undertake. You want a diet that leaves you feeling energized, with enough mojo to tackle that big project at work, the renovation of your house, the half-marathon you're training for, or dealing with the demands of your toddler.

Falling off the Wagon (and Climbing Back up Again)

In my next life, I am going to be perfect from the word "go." Bed made every morning, floss every night, meditate 20 minutes daily, read *The New Yorker* instead of *People* magazine, volunteer with the elderly, never lose my temper, and refuse to allow a bad hair day to affect my self-worth.

That's the next go-round. In this life, things are different. I do manage to make the bed every day and floss five (okay, four) nights a week, but I throw money at social issues instead of volunteering my time and have more than once been found sobbing in the ladies room, only minutes before a client meeting, clutching a hair straightener in one hand and smoothing gel in the other in a desperate attempt to get rid of the frizzies.

First-world problems, I know. But stay with me on this one. How we handle the smaller issues of life are a reflection of our mental sturdiness and emotional toughness to weather the bigger storms.

For example, I know I lean toward the "all-or-nothing" mentality. It's why I do endurance sports. If I'm going to run, I'm going to run—a *lot*. Same thing with cycling or weight lifting. If I muster the resolve to show up to work out, then let's throw out the excuses and get to work. Otherwise it's a waste of the mental effort it took to get me up, dressed, and out the door in the first place.

I bring the same attitude to my diet. I want it to be all or nothing. Because of that, I'm often harsh in my criticism of myself when I don't achieve the perfection of which I believe I am capable. I may eat perfectly for three days and do nothing more than have a rice cake (a rice cake!) with almond butter one day as a snack and allow that one small lapse to snowball into a full-blown "Who am I and why do I even try?" mental breakdown. Which, as we all know, leads to even more poor eating choices.

Here's the thing. Following the 80/20 principle, there is nothing wrong with the occasional lapse so long as the occasional lapse doesn't turn into the "once a day" and then the "twice a day" and then the "I ate a PV breakfast so I'll cheat at lunch" lapse.

What kind of mental fortitude do you carry? Can you drink a vanilla soy latte and do a quick rebound to get back on track or do you allow the smallest falter to throw you off your game and spiral you into an unhealthy cycle of eating? Because here's the thing: At some point, the odds are strong you'll fall off the PV wagon. Whether you down a Greek yogurt or a full quart of Ben & Jerry's raw chocolate-chip cookie dough ice cream (go big or go home, I always say), what matters isn't that you ate the non-PV food. What matters is how you bounce back.

Ideally, you'll recognize the event for what it was: a momentary lapse that, contrary to what you may be thinking, does *not* say volumes about who you are as a person. Mistakes happen. Some not of your own doing. You may unintentionally stumble when you're invited to a friend's house for dinner and you later discover the vegetables they made especially for you were cooked in canola oil. Just last week my mom left a Tupperware container for me in the fridge packed with a batch of slow cooker vegetables she'd made just for me. I gobbled down the tender carrots, mushrooms, cauliflower, and onions. I called my mom to thank her for the food.

"Delicious!" I said. "What was that sauce it was covered in?"

"A1 Steak Sauce."

I ran to the computer and Googled, "A1 Steak Sauce[35] ingredients," already knowing the answer. Yup, right there on the screen. Made with corn syrup. Four grams of sugar per tablespoon. God only knows how many tablespoons of the stuff my mom dumped in there, thinking that because it was only vegetables, she was making me a Paleo Vegetarian meal.

The point is, you're not Superman with x-ray vision into the kitchen of every friend's home. It would have been easy for me to get down about "ruining" my diet with the sugar and corn syrup (and the caramel color, potassium sorbate, and xanthan gum) in the A1, but I cut myself the necessary slack to shrug it off. It also would have been easy to get upset with my mom—who knows I follow a Paleo diet and has been lectured by me 1,001 times on what is and is not allowed and that she needs to *check ingredients* before she feeds me—for dousing the vegetables in the stuff and putting it in my fridge. But the bottom line is blame and guilt don't get anyone anywhere. Instead of moving into an "I hate myself for doing that" soliloquy, I chose instead to focus on the fact that most of what I

---

35 By the way, there are plenty of yummy PV substitutions for A1 Steak Sauce. Combining tomato paste, olive oil, and balsamic vinegar with crushed garlic and a smidge of cayenne pepper is a favorite of mine, or just Google "Paleo steak sauce." Ignore the ones that use the fat bastings from meat as the base, and boom, you're in business.

ate was vegetables. And that my mom loves me enough to cook for me and leave me food as a gift. That's nothing to sneeze at.

Eating a sauce that you later discover has a little soy in it is a lot different from mindlessly scarfing down a flour-based, gooey cheese pizza. Both may happen. It's life. You're not meant to be perfect. Give yourself a pep talk, climb back on board the PV wagon, and keep moving forward.

With PV as a foundation for health, life is only going to keep getting better.

Chapter 18

The Final Analysis: Is PV the Right Diet for Me?

Now that you've read about the good, the bad, and the yummy, it's decision time. Is this the right diet for you?

For better or worse, food is a big part of who we are. Our family and social lives often revolve around it. It's the trigger for how we feel about our health, our bodies, and ourselves. It impacts everything from the way we think to the physical activities in which we choose to engage. For that reason, it's worth taking some time to think about how we want to live. Not just "I want to be thin," but also "How am I going to think about and relate to food for the rest of my life?"

That's kind of a big deal. And it's why, unlike other diet books that claim, "Yes! This is the perfect diet for everyone!" I'm okay with putting it out there that a Paleo Vegetarian diet is *not* for everyone. There probably isn't a diet out there that you can't lose weight on, assuming you can hang with the rules. But diets that rely on calorie restriction and leave us feeling hungry and deprived rarely work. At least, not long-term. The Paleo Vegetarian diet is simple in that you eat whole, nutritious foods that nurture your body, fill you up, and make you feel good. It's a challenge, however, because we live in a society that relies on prepackaged, fast-food convenience, and Paleo Vegetarianism doesn't fall into that box.

You may think you know just from reading this book whether Paleo Vegetarianism is a sustainable way of eating for you. However, the very fact that you picked up this book indicates food, your health, and your diet are important factors in how you chose to live your life. For that reason, even if you're undecided, give it a whirl. The best (and really, only) way to determine if this way of engaging with food works for you, your lifestyle, and your goals is to commit to a time period—one month, three months, six months—and see how it goes. Measure your results in inches lost, your energy level, and how you feel. Chances are, once you start, you're not going to recognize the soft, sluggish, carbohydrate-overdosed individual you used to be.

However, let's play fair. Below are some areas to monitor as you move forward with the PV plan. These areas are hurdles most people switching to a PV diet deal with. There are ways to move through each of them, but it may be you find yourself stuck in one or more. If you can't move past them, it may make sense for you to consider a different way of eating. Don't jump to conclusions, but do keep these areas in mind and use them as a basis for evaluating whether or not the Paleo Vegetarian diet is right for you.

MORE ENERGY. Any diet that leaves you feeling lethargic and drained won't work long-term. Assuming you've made it past the carb-flu stage, you should be experiencing a noticeable increase in your energy levels. This is the transition from being a sugar-burning to a fat-burning beast that we've discussed. If after months of eating PV you find yourself drained and tired, something's off. It may be you're not getting enough carbs, protein, or healthy fats.

Make some adjustments to see if adding more carbs like sweet potatoes or more protein does the trick.

NO TIME TO COOK. Maybe you've identified you're not getting enough protein or healthy fats. But if the problem is your schedule doesn't allow you the time to plan and cook to get the balance of foods you need for your body to feel good, this may not be the diet for you. Cut yourself some slack on this, though, before you make this a reason to leave the plan. It takes time to establish cooking and go-to recipe routines. Once you know what to eat, cooking your PV meals truly does go a whole lot faster.

GAUGING HUNGER. I refuse to go through life hungry and you should too. Simply put, it's just a miserable way to live. If you find yourself constantly hungry on the PV diet, you're doing it wrong. (See how I put the blame on you, not me? I'm so clever.) Fortunately, the fix is simple: Eat more. While PV is not a free-for-all food fest, the fact that you're eating whole, natural foods that are heavy on vegetables means you can—and should—eat enough to satiate your hunger. There is no calorie counting, and as long as you're keeping your sugar intake low, you can eat to your satisfaction and still lose weight. The key here is learning to differentiate between true hunger and the sneakier "Ooh, that sounds good and I want some" hankerings. Listen to your body and let it tell you if you're really hungry or if it's just an in-the-moment craving.

FEELING DEPRIVED. There's a difference between feeling hungry and feeling deprived. Hunger is a physical need. Feeling deprived is a mental/emotional aspect that often accompanies changing our diet. It's normal to feel deprived at the start of a diet that requires a major change in your eating patterns. That's why the Paleo blogs are filled with people reminiscing about pancakes. You may have experienced a feeling of deprivation when you went vegetarian and your plate suddenly looked empty without the big portion of meat or fish to fill it up. But once you adjust to the lifestyle and find your way around the foods and new meals you'll create, that feeling of deprivation should subside. If it doesn't, take a closer look at why not. Are you eating enough fat and protein to fill you up? Are you still seeing food as a reward or punishment instead of as a nourishment for your body? Are you "cheating" a little too often, not allowing your body to transform from sugar burning to fat burning and therefore keeping the sugar cravings in place? If you're consistently feeling deprived, it's worth tracking your food intake and mood for at least a week to see if you can pinpoint what's triggering these feelings, allowing you to find workarounds to overcome them.

LOSING INCHES AND FEELING FIRMER. It's hard to step away from the scale but please, please try. It's such an arbitrary number; especially as good, healthy (sexy!) muscles weigh more than even being skinny-fat. Instead of judging progress by a number, take your measurements or a photo before you start PV and then revisit on a monthly basis moving forward and judge results that way. Wouldn't you rather be a firm, sculpted 145 pounds versus a soft, bloated, and jiggly 130? The PV diet isn't about tricks or quick water-weight loss. We're after long-term sustainable health that empowers your body to conquer whatever you place before it. Badass takes time. Keep that in mind.

ALIENATING FRIENDS AND FAMILY. There's no question that eating PV is going to set you apart from friends and family, at least in terms of what you eat. Sometimes, there are greater consequences. A spouse might apply pressure or guilt about why you can't eat what the family eats. Coworkers may gently (or not so gently) mock you. You may grow tired of the raised eyebrows or having to explain yet again what you do and don't eat and your reasons behind it. All of this can cause stress. And too much stress can wreak havoc on even the best-laid plans for our bodies. If you're constantly fighting battles and feeling like your diet is coming between you and the people you love, maybe this isn't the plan for you—at least right now. But that doesn't mean you can't take portions of what you've learned (limit the grains and sugar) and apply it until you're in a better place to circle back around and go all-in.

HOW DO YOU FEEL? Ultimately, the best measure of any diet is how it makes you feel. Do you feel stronger, healthier, and more energized? Do you feel your body responding in a positive manner to the changes you're making? Do you feel proud of yourself for taking care of your body and mind, and laying the foundation for a healthy future? Do you enjoy the foods you're eating? While the answer may not be "yes!" 100 percent of the time, it should be "yes" more often than not. We eat to feel healthy, happy, and strong. Make sure your way of eating makes you feel that way.

Putting It All Together

Ultimately, there is no one "right" or "wrong" way to eat. Different paths work for different people. Just make sure that before you undertake this or any diet you have an understanding of why you're choosing to eat a certain way, what your goals are, what you hope to accomplish, and why you think this is the plan that will get you there. No leaps of faith, no surprises. Instead, opt for a rational, well-thought-out path where you're aware of obstacles and have made plans to overcome them.

This is your body and your life. Make the choices that are right for you.

Happy PV eating!

—Dena

Conversion Charts

Temperature Conversions

FAHRENHEIT (°F)	CELSIUS (°C)
325°F	165°C
350°F	175°C
375°F	190°C
400°F	200°C
425°F	220°C
450°F	230°C

Volume Conversions

U.S.	U.S. EQUIVALENT	METRIC
1 tablespoon (3 teaspoons)	½ fluid ounce	15 milliliters
¼ cup	2 fluid ounces	60 milliliters
⅓ cup	3 fluid ounces	90 milliliters
½ cup	4 fluid ounces	120 milliliters
⅔ cup	5 fluid ounces	150 milliliters
¾ cup	6 fluid ounces	180 milliliters
1 cup	8 fluid ounces	240 milliliters
2 cups	16 fluid ounces	480 milliliters

Weight Conversions

U.S.	METRIC
½ ounce	15 grams
1 ounce	30 grams
2 ounces	60 grams
¼ pound	115 grams
⅓ pound	150 grams
½ pound	225 grams
¾ pound	350 grams
1 pound	450 grams

Index

About the Author

Dena Harris is a writer, author, and endurance athlete living in North Carolina. She is also an ambitious if not entirely trustworthy cook. Dena is the author of numerous gift/humor books about cats, including the internationally sold *Who Moved My Mouse? A Self-Help Book for Cats (Who Don't Need Any Help)*. A former couch potato, Dena has completed 15 marathons—including two Bostons—and a handful of ultras. She is training for her first Ironman. For more information on Dena, her books, and a chance to read a riveting description on her blog of what she recently ate for lunch, visit DenaHarris.com.